CONTENTS

VEGETABLE & VEGETARIAN RECIPES 6

Wood Pellet Grilled Asparagus And Honey Glazed Carrots 6

Grilled Asparagus With Wild Mushrooms 6

Spinach Soup 6

Southern Slaw 6

Roasted Peach Salsa 7

Ramen Soup 7

Smoked Healthy Cabbage 7

Wood Pellet Smoked Asparagus 8

Crispy Maple Bacon Brussels Sprouts 8

Smoked 3-bean Salad 8

Vegan Smoked Carrot Dogs 8

Apple Veggie Burger 9

Roasted Hasselback Potatoes 9

Bunny Dogs With Sweet And Spicy Jalapeño Relish 9

Caldereta Stew 10

Roasted Parmesan Cheese Broccoli 10

Smoked Baked Beans 11

Grilled Ratatouille Salad 11

Wood Pellet Bacon Wrapped Jalapeno Poppers 11

Smoked Balsamic Potatoes And Carrots 11

Kale Chips 12

Garlic And Rosemary Potato Wedges 12

Smoked Deviled Eggs 12

Fries With Chipotle Ketchup 13

Roasted Root Vegetables 13

Smoked Pumpkin Soup 13

Wood Pellet Smoked Vegetables 14

Grilled Corn On The Cob With Parmesan And Garlic 14

Sweet Potato Chips 14

Roasted Butternut Squash 15

Potato Fries With Chipotle Peppers 15

Garlic And Herb Smoke Potato 15

Grilled Zucchini Squash 16

Minestrone Soup 16

Baked Parmesan Mushrooms 16

Grilled Zucchini Squash Spears 17

Roasted Veggies & Hummus 17

Smoked Potato Salad 17

Wood Pellet Smoked Acorn Squash 17

Mexican Street Corn With Chipotle Butter 2 18

Roasted Okra 18

Sweet Potato Fries 18

Grilled Cherry Tomato Skewers 19

Georgia Sweet Onion Bake 19

Salt-crusted Baked Potatoes 19

Whole Roasted Cauliflower With Garlic Parmesan Butter 20

Bacon-wrapped Jalapeño Poppers 20

Roasted Spicy Tomatoes 20

Shiitake Smoked Mushrooms 20

Smoked Eggs 21

Coconut Bacon 21

Grilled Broccoli 21

Smoked Baked Kale Chips 21

Smokey Roasted Cauliflower 22

Baked Sweet And Savory Yams 22

Smoked Mushrooms 22

Smoked And Smashed New Potatoes 23

Butter Braised Green Beans 23

Stuffed Grilled Zucchini 23

Grilled Asparagus & Honey-glazed Carrots 23

Roasted Vegetable Medley 24

Corn Chowder 24

Carolina Baked Beans 24

POULTRY RECIPES 26

Glazed Chicken Thighs 26

Authentic Holiday Turkey Breast 26

Lemon Rosemary And Beer Marinated Chicken 26

Herb Roasted Turkey 27

Lemon Chicken Breast 27

Peach And Basil Grilled Chicken 27

Beer Can–smoked Chicken 28

Rosemary Orange Chicken 28

Smo-fried Chicken 29

Wood Pellet Smoked Spatchcock Turkey 29

Special Occasion's Dinner Cornish Hen 29

Peppered Bbq Chicken Thighs 30

Jamaican Jerk Chicken Quarters 30

Christmas Dinner Goose 30

Crispy & Juicy Chicken 31

Grill Bbq Chicken Breasts 31

Smoked Turkey Breast 32

Easy Smoked Chicken Breasts 32

Wood Pellet Sheet Pan Chicken Fajitas 32

Asian Miso Chicken Wings........................ 32

Beer Can Chicken.. 33

Roasted Whole Chicken 33

Garlic Parmesan Chicken Wings.............. 33

Honey Garlic Chicken Wings.................... 34

Wood Pellet Grilled Buffalo Chicken Leg.......... 34

Wood Pellet Smoked Spatchcock Turkey......... 34

Chili Barbecue Chicken 34

Wood Pellet Grilled Chicken 35

Hickory Smoked Chicken 35

Smoked Turkey Wings 35

Wild Turkey Egg Rolls 36

Grilled Buffalo Chicken Legs 36

Wood Pellet Chicken Breasts.................... 36

Buttered Thanksgiving Turkey.................. 37

Buffalo Chicken Wraps 37

Smoking Duck With Mandarin Glaze.............. 38

Turkey Meatballs.. 38

Smoked Lemon Chicken Breasts.............. 38

Smoked Fried Chicken................................ 39

Buffalo Chicken Flatbread........................ 39

Cinco De Mayo Chicken Enchiladas 39

Sweet And Spicy Smoked Wings 40

Cajun Chicken... 40

Turkey Breast.. 40

Rustic Maple Smoked Chicken Wings 41

Sheet Pan Chicken Fajitas 41

Chinese Inspired Duck Legs 41

Paprika Chicken 42

Grilled Chicken 42

Perfectly Smoked Turkey Legs 42

Chicken Wings 43

Turkey With Apricot Barbecue Glaze............... 43

Smoked Whole Duck 43

Maple And Bacon Chicken........................ 44

Bbq Sauce Smothered Chicken Breasts........... 44

Wood Pellet Smoked Cornish Hens.................. 44

Wood Pellet Chile Lime Chicken 45

Hickory Smoked Chicken Leg And Thigh

Quarters.. 45

Buffalo Wings 45

Spatchcocked Turkey................................. 45

Wood-fired Chicken Breasts 46

Hot And Sweet Spatchcocked Chicken............ 46

Wild West Wings.. 46

BEEF,PORK & LAMB RECIPES 48

Bbq Sweet Pepper Meatloaf 48

St. Louis Bbq Ribs 48

The Perfect T-bones................................... 48

Pork Steak... 49

Wood Pellet Smoked Leg Of lamb..................... 49

Reverse Seared Flank Steak 49

Trager New York Strip............................... 50

Pork Belly.. 50

Pineapple Pork Bbq 50

Braised Elk Shank...................................... 51

Country Pork Roast.................................... 51

Wood Pellet Togarashi Pork Tenderloin 51

Texas Smoked Brisket................................ 52

Chinese Bbq Pork....................................... 52

Real Treat Chuck Roast 53

Wood Pellet Grilled Shredded Pork Tacos....... 53

Smoked And Pulled Beef........................... 53

Cowboy Steak... 53

Citrus-brined Pork Roast.......................... 54

Smoked Pork Sausages.............................. 54

Beef Shoulder Clod 55

Strip Steak With Onion Sauce................... 55

Grilled Cuban Pork Chops 55

Garlic Rack Of Lamb.................................. 56

Versatile Beef Tenderloin......................... 56

Pineapple-pepper Pork Kebabs 57

Beef Jerky.. 57

Smoked, Candied, And Spicy Bacon 57

Elegant Lamb Chops.................................. 58

Lamb Shank.. 58

Mesquite Smoked Brisket 58

Bbq Baby Back Ribs................................... 59

Sweet & Spicy Pork Roast......................... 59

Stunning Prime Rib Roast......................... 60

Citrus Pork Chops 60

Southern Sugar-glazed Ham.................... 60

Slow Roasted Shawarma 61

Cowboy Cut Steak...................................... 61

Braised Lamb.. 62

Drunken Beef Jerky.................................... 62

Spicy & Tangy Lamb Shoulder 62

Kalbi Beef Ribs... 63

French Onion Burgers................................ 63

Sweet Smoked Country Ribs 64

Cocoa Crusted Pork Tenderloin............... 64

Smoked Pork Tenderloin........................... 64

Wood Pellet Grilled Lamb With Brown Sugar

Glaze.. 65

Smoked Sausages..65
Bbq Brisket...65
Asian Steak Skewers..66
Bacon..66
Smoked Lamb Meatballs.................................66
Bbq Breakfast Grits..67
Braised Short Ribs..67
Wood Pellet Grill Pork Crown Roast.................68
Smoked Longhorn Cowboy Tri-tip....................68
Smoked Pork Ribs 68
Rosemary Lamb 68
Stuffed Peppers 69
Braised Mediterranean Beef Brisket.................69
Greek-style Roast Leg Of Lamb.........................70
Chili Rib Eye Steaks 70
Santa Maria Tri-tip...71

FISH AND SEAFOOD RECIPES...................72
Sriracha Salmon 72
Lobster Tail 72
Togarashi Smoked Salmon 72
Stuffed Shrimp Tilapia......................................73
Lobster Tails 73
Wood Pellet Togarashi Grilled Salmon.............74
Charleston Crab Cakes With Remoulade.........74
Dijon-smoked Halibut.......................................74
Citrus Salmon 75
Bacon-wrapped Shrimp....................................75
Juicy Smoked Salmon......................................75
Smoked Shrimp 76
Grilled Blackened Salmon 76
Lemon Garlic Scallops......................................76
Pacific Northwest Salmon 77
Grilled Shrimp Kabobs 77
Oysters In The Shell..77
Super-tasty Trout 77
Flavor-bursting Prawn Skewers 78
Grilled Tilapia..78
Cajun-blackened Shrimp 78
Grilled Shrimp Scampi.....................................79
Wood Pellet Salt And Pepper Spot Prawn
Skewers 79
Wine Infused Salmon.......................................79
Lively Flavored Shrimp......................................80
Grilled Lingcod...80
Lobster Tail 80
Salmon With Togarashi.....................................80
Bacon-wrapped Scallops 81

Cod With Lemon Herb Butter...............................81
Summer Paella...81
Cider Salmon...82
Wood Pellet Rockfish 82
Cajun Catfish 83
Grilled King Crab Legs 83
No-fuss Tuna Burgers..83
Wood Pellet Teriyaki Smoked Shrimp.................83
Mussels With Pancetta Aïoli...............................84
Grilled Lingcod...84
Smoked Shrimp 85
Salmon With Avocado Salsa 85
Crazy Delicious Lobster Tails 85
Omega-3 Rich Salmon..85
Enticing Mahi-mahi...86
Grilled Tuna 86
Grilled Salmon...86
Fish Fillets With Pesto 87
Grilled Rainbow Trout..87
Cajun Seasoned Shrimp......................................87
Jerk Shrimp..87
Teriyaki Smoked Shrimp......................................88
Wood Pellet Garlic Dill Smoked Salmon............88
Chilean Sea Bass 88
Grilled Shrimp 89
Mango Shrimp 89
Cajun Smoked Catfish 89
Grilled Lobster Tail 90
Hot-smoked Salmon..90
Halibut With Garlic Pesto.....................................90
Buttered Crab Legs..91
Spicy Shrimps Skewers 91
Seared Tuna Steaks...91
Wood Pellet Smoked Salmon...............................92

OTHER FAVORITE RECIPES................................. 93
Smoked Cheese Dip...93
Smoked Pork Ribs With Fresh Herbs 93
Chile Cheeseburgers..93
Smoked Chuck Roast..94
Cold Hot Smoked Salmon 94
Curried Chicken Roast With Tarragon And
Custard 94
Smoked Bananas Foster Bread Pudding............95
Seafood On Skewers..95
Smoked Garlic White Sauce................................96
Garlic Aioli And Smoked Salmon Sliders...........96
Smoked Chicken With Perfect Poultry Rub 96

Pizza Bianca 97
Barbecue Sandwich 97
Reverse-seared Tilapia 98
Cornish Game Hens 98
Black Bean Dipping Sauce 98
Roasted Ham 98
Polish Kielbasa 99
Super-addicting Mushrooms 99
Pork Fennel Burger 99
Spiced Nuts 100
Grilled Bacon Dog 100
Roasted Almonds 100
Steak Sauce 101
Native Southern Cornbread 101
Buttered Green Peas 101
Twice-baked Spaghetti Squash 102
Avocado Smoothie 102
Pan-seared Pork Tenderloin With Apple
Mashed Potatoes 102
Smoked Teriyaki Tuna 103
Sweet Sensation Pork Meat 103

Hickory Smoked Green Beans 103
Banana Walnut Bread 104
Empanadas 104
Cumin Salt 105
Marinated Chicken Kabobs 105
Potluck Favorite Baked Beans 105
Red Wine Beef Stew 106
Seafaring Seafood Rub With Smoked
Swordfish 106
Smoked Tuna 106
Wood Pellet Spicy Brisket 107
Banana Nut Oatmeal 107
Pork Carnitas 107
Baked Wild Sockeye Salmon 108
Baby Bok Choy With Lime-miso Vinaigrette 108
Turkey Sandwich 108
Smoked Spicy Pork Medallions 109
Monster Smoked Pork Chops 109
APPENDIX : RECIPES INDEX 110

VEGETABLE & VEGETARIAN RECIPES

Wood Pellet Grilled Asparagus And Honey Glazed Carrots

Servings: 5
Cooking Time: 35 Minutes
Ingredients:

- 1 bunch asparagus, trimmed ends
- 1 lb carrots, peeled
- 2 tbsp olive oil
- Sea salt to taste
- 2 tbsp honey
- Lemon zest

Directions:

1. Sprinkle the asparagus with oil and sea salt. Drizzle the carrots with honey and salt.
2. Preheat the wood pellet to 165°F wit the lid closed for 15 minutes.
3. Place the carrots in the wood pellet and cook for 15 minutes. Add asparagus and cook for 20 more minutes or until cooked through.
4. Top the carrots and asparagus with lemon zest. Enjoy.

Nutrition Info: Calories 1680, Total fat 30g, Saturated fat 2g, Total Carbs 10g, Net Carbs 10g, Protein 4g, Sugar 0g, Fiber 0g, Sodium: 514mg, Potassium 0mg

Grilled Asparagus With Wild Mushrooms

Servings: 4
Cooking Time: 10 Minutes
Ingredients:

- 2 bunches fresh asparagus, trimmed
- 4 cups wild mushrooms, sliced
- 1 large shallots, sliced into rings
- Extra virgin oil as needed
- 2 tablespoons butter, melted

Directions:

1. Fire the Grill to 500F. Use desired wood pellets when cooking. Close the lid and preheat for 15 minutes.
2. Place the asparagus, mushrooms, and shallots on a baking tray. Drizzle with oil and butter and season with salt and pepper to taste.

3. Place on a baking tray and cook for 10 minutes. Make sure to give the asparagus a good stir halfway through the cooking time for even browning.

Nutrition Info: Calories per serving: 218; Protein: 15.2g; Carbs: 26.6 g; Fat: 10g Sugar: 12.9g

Spinach Soup

Servings: 4
Cooking Time: 35 Minutes
Ingredients:

- 2cups Chicken Stock
- 2tbsp. Vegetable Oil
- 1Onion quartered
- 2 ½ cup Spinach
- ½ lb. Red Potatoes, sliced thinly
- 2cups Milk, whole
- 1Leek, large and sliced thinly
- Black Pepper and Sea Salt, as needed
- 1Thyme Sprigs
- 1Bay Leaf

Directions:

1. For making this healthy soup, place the oil, onion, bay leaf, and thyme in the blender pitcher.
2. Now, press the 'saute' button.
3. Once sautéed, stir in the rest of the ingredients and press the 'smooth soup' button.
4. Finally, transfer the soup to the serving bowls and serve it hot.

Nutrition Info: Calories: 403 Fat: 24 g Total Carbs: 32 g Fiber: 3 g Sugar: 5.5 g Protein: 15 g Cholesterol: 66 mg

Southern Slaw

Servings: 10
Cooking Time: 1 Hour And 10 Minutes
Ingredients:

- 1 head cabbage, shredded
- ¼ cup white vinegar
- ¼ cup sugar
- 1 teaspoon paprika
- ½ teaspoon salt
- ½ teaspoon freshly ground black pepper

- 1 cup heavy (whipping) cream

Directions:

1. Place the shredded cabbage in a large bowl.
2. In a small bowl, combine the vinegar, sugar, paprika, salt, and pepper.
3. Pour the vinegar mixture over the cabbage and mix well.
4. Fold in the heavy cream and refrigerate for at least 1 hour before serving.

Roasted Peach Salsa

Servings: 6
Cooking Time: 10 Minutes
Ingredients:

- 6 whole peaches, pitted and halved
- 3 tomatoes, chopped
- 2 whole onions, chopped
- ½ cup cilantro, chopped
- 2 cloves garlic, minced
- 5 teaspoons apple cider vinegar
- ½ teaspoon salt
- ¼ teaspoon black pepper
- 2 tablespoons olive oil

Directions:

1. Fire the Grill to 300F. Use desired wood pellets when cooking. Close the lid and preheat for 15 minutes.
2. Place the peaches on the grill grate and cook for 5 minutes on each side. Remove from the grill and allow to rest for 5 minutes.
3. Place the peaches, tomatoes, onion, and cilantro in a salad bowl. On a smaller bowl, stir in the garlic, apple cider vinegar, salt, pepper, and olive oil. Stir until well-combined. Pour into the salad and toss to coat.

Nutrition Info: Calories per serving: 155 ;
Protein: 3.1g; Carbs: 27.6 g; Fat: 5.1g Sugar: 20g

Ramen Soup

Servings: 2
Cooking Time: 35 Minutes
Ingredients:

- 4cups Chicken Stock
- 1tbsp. Extra Virgin Olive Oil

- 2Baby Bok Choy Head, leaves torn
- 1Shallot, chopped into 1-inch piece
- 3oz. Ramen, dried
- 4Garlic cloves
- 1tsp. Sesame Oil, toasted
- 2tsp. Ginger, fresh
- One bunch of Green Onion, sliced thinly
- 1cup Chicken, cooked and cut into 1-inch cubes

Directions:

1. First, keep the olive oil, shallot, garlic, and ginger in the blender pitcher.
2. After that, press the 'saute' button.
3. Next, stir in the chicken, green onions, chicken stock, and sesame oil into it.
4. Now, select the 'hearty soup' button.
5. Then, three minutes before the program ends, spoon in the ramen noodles and baby bok choy.
6. Check the chicken's internal temperature and ensure it is 165 ° F and if it is, then transfer the soup to the serving bowls.
7. Serve immediately and enjoy it.

Nutrition Info: Calories: 190 Fat: 8g Total Carbs: 25g Fiber: 1 g Sugar: 0.5 g Protein: 3 g Cholesterol: 2.5 mg

Smoked Healthy Cabbage

Servings: 5
Cooking Time: 2 Hours
Ingredients:

- 1head cabbage, cored
- 4tablespoons butter
- 2tablespoons rendered bacon fat
- 1chicken bouillon cube
- 1teaspoon fresh ground black pepper
- 1garlic clove, minced

Directions:

1. Preheat your smoker to 240 degrees Fahrenheit using your preferred wood
2. Fill the hole of your cored cabbage with butter, bouillon cube, bacon fat, pepper and garlic
3. Wrap the cabbage in foil about two-thirds of the way up
4. Make sure to leave the top open
5. Transfer to your smoker rack and smoke for 2 hours
6. Unwrap and enjoy!

Nutrition Info: Calories: 231 Fats: 10g Carbs: 26g Fiber: 1g

Wood Pellet Smoked Asparagus

Servings: 4
Cooking Time: 1 Hour
Ingredients:
- 1 bunch fresh asparagus, ends cut
- 2 tbsp olive oil
- Salt and pepper to taste

Directions:
1. Fire up your wood pellet smoker to 230°F
2. Place the asparagus in a mixing bowl and drizzle with olive oil. Season with salt and pepper.
3. Place the asparagus in a tinfoil sheet and fold the sides such that you create a basket.
4. Smoke the asparagus for 1 hour or until soft turning after half an hour.
5. Remove from the grill and serve. Enjoy.

Nutrition Info: Calories 43, Total fat 2g, Saturated fat 0g, Total Carbs 4g, Net Carbs 2g, Protein 3g, Sugar 2g, Fiber 2g, Sodium: 148mg

Crispy Maple Bacon Brussels Sprouts

Servings: 6
Cooking Time: 1 Hour
Ingredients:
- 1lb brussels sprouts, trimmed and quartered
- 6 slices thick-cut bacon
- 3tbsp maple syrup
- 1tsp olive oil
- 1/2 tsp kosher salt
- 1/2 tsp ground black pepper

Directions:
1. Preheat pellet grill to 425°F.
2. Cut bacon into 1/2 inch thick slices.
3. Place brussels sprouts in a single layer in the cast iron skillet. Drizzle with olive oil and maple syrup, then toss to coat. Sprinkle bacon slices on top then season with kosher salt and black pepper.
4. Place skillet in the pellet grill and roast for about 40 to 45 minutes, or until the brussels sprouts are caramelized and brown.

5. Remove skillet from grill and allow brussels sprouts to cool for about 5 to 10 minutes. Serve and enjoy!

Nutrition Info: Calories: 175.3 Fat: 12.1 g Cholesterol: 6.6 mg Carbohydrate: 13.6 g Fiber: 2.9 g Sugar: 7.6 g Protein: 4.8 g

Smoked 3-bean Salad

Servings: 6
Cooking Time: 20 Minutes
Ingredients:
- 1 can Great Northern Beans, rinsed and drained
- 1 can Red Kidney Beans, rinsed and drained
- 1pound fresh green beans, trimmed
- 2 tablespoons olive oil
- Salt and pepper to taste
- 1 shallot, sliced thinly
- 2 tablespoons red wine vinegar
- 1 teaspoon Dijon mustard

Directions:
1. Fire the Grill to 500F. Use desired wood pellets when cooking. Close the lid and preheat for 15 minutes.
2. Place the beans in a sheet tray and drizzle with olive oil. Season with salt and pepper to taste.
3. Place in the grill and cook for 20 minutes. Make sure to shake the tray for even cooking.
4. Once cooked, remove the beans and place in a bowl. Allow to cool first.
5. Add the shallots and the rest of the ingredients. Season with more salt and pepper if desired. Toss to coat the beans with the seasoning.

Nutrition Info: Calories per serving: 179; Protein: 8.2 g; Carbs: 23.5g; Fat: 6.5g Sugar: 2.2g

Vegan Smoked Carrot Dogs

Servings: 2
Cooking Time: 35 Minutes
Ingredients:
- 4 carrots, thick
- 2 tbsp avocado oil
- 1/2 tbsp garlic powder
- 1 tbsp liquid smoke
- Pepper to taste

- Kosher salt to taste

Directions:

1. Preheat your to 425F then line a parchment paper on a baking sheet.
2. Peel the carrots to resemble a hot dog. Round the edges when peeling.
3. Whisk together oil, garlic powder, liquid smoke, pepper and salt in a bowl, small.
4. Now place carrots on the baking sheet and pour the mixture over. Roll your carrots in the mixture to massage seasoning and oil into them. Use fingertips.
5. Roast the carrots in the until fork tender for about 35 minutes. Brush the carrots using the marinade mixture every 5 minutes.
6. Remove and place into hot dog buns then top with hot dog toppings of your choice.
7. Serve and enjoy!

Nutrition Info: Calories 76, Total fat 1.8g, Saturated 0.4g, Total 14.4g, Net carbs 10.6g, Protein 1.5g, Sugar 6.6g, Fiber 3.8g, Sodium 163mg, Potassium 458mg

Apple Veggie Burger

Servings: 6
Cooking Time: 35 Minutes
Ingredients:

- 3 tbsp ground flax or ground chia
- 1/3 cup of warm water
- 1/2 cups rolled oats
- 1 cup chickpeas, drained and rinsed
- 1 tsp cumin
- 1/2 cup onion
- 1 tsp dried basil
- 2 granny smith apples
- 1/3 cup parsley or cilantro, chopped
- 2 tbsp soy sauce
- 2 tsp liquid smoke
- 2 cloves garlic, minced
- 1 tsp chili powder
- 1/4 tsp black pepper

Directions:

1. Preheat the smoker to 225°F while adding wood chips and water to it.
2. In a separate bowl, add chickpeas and mash. Mix together the remaining ingredients along with the dipped flax seeds.

3. Form patties from this mixture.
4. Put the patties on the rack of the smoker and smoke them for 20 minutes on each side.
5. When brown, take them out, and serve.

Nutrition Info: Calories: 241 Cal Fat: 5 g Carbohydrates: 40 g   Protein: 9 g Fiber: 10.3 g

Roasted Hasselback Potatoes

Servings: 6
Cooking Time: 30 Minutes
Ingredients:

- 6 large russet potatoes
- 1-pound bacon
- ½ cup butter
- Salt to taste
- 1 cup cheddar cheese
- 3 whole scallions, chopped

Directions:

1. Fire the Grill to 350F. Use desired wood pellets when cooking. Close the lid and preheat for 15 minutes.
2. Place two wooden spoons on either side of the potato and slice the potato into thin strips without completely cutting through the potato.
3. Chop the bacon into small pieces and place in between the cracks or slices of the potatoes.
4. Place potatoes in a cast iron skillet. Top the potatoes with butter, salt, and cheddar cheese.
5. Place the skillet on the grill grate and cook for 30 minutes. Make sure to baste the potatoes with melted cheese 10 minutes before the cooking time ends.

Nutrition Info: Calories per serving: 662; Protein: 16.1g; Carbs: 71.5g; Fat: 38g Sugar: 2.3g

Bunny Dogs With Sweet And Spicy Jalapeño Relish

Servings: 8
Cooking Time: 35 To 40 Minutes
Ingredients:

- 8 hot dog-size carrots, peeled
- ¼ cup honey
- ¼ cup yellow mustard
- Nonstick cooking spray or butter, for greasing

- Salt
- Freshly ground black pepper
- 8 hot dog buns
- Sweet and Spicy Jalapeño Relish

Directions:

1. Prepare the carrots by removing the stems and slicing in half lengthwise.
2. In a small bowl, whisk together the honey and mustard.
3. Supply your smoker with wood pellets and follow the manufacturer's specific start-up procedure. Preheat, with the lid closed, to 375°F.
4. Line a baking sheet with aluminum foil and coat with cooking spray.
5. Brush the carrots on both sides with the honey mustard and season with salt and pepper; put on the baking sheet.
6. Place the baking sheet on the grill grate, close the lid, and smoke for 35 to 40 minutes, or until tender and starting to brown.
7. To serve, lightly toast the hot dog buns on the grill and top each with two slices of carrot and some relish.

Caldereta Stew

Servings: 12

Cooking Time: 4 Hours

Ingredients:

- 2lb. chuck roast, sliced into cubes
- 2tablespoons olive oil
- 1carrot, sliced into cubes
- 2potatoes, sliced into cubes
- 4garlic cloves, chopped
- 2tablespoons tomato paste
- 2cups tomato sauce
- 2red bell peppers, sliced into strips
- 2green bell peppers, sliced into strips
- 2cups of water
- 1/2 cup cheddar cheese, grated
- 1/4 cup liver spread
- Salt to taste

Directions:

1. Put the beef in a cast iron pan.
2. Place this in the smoking cabinet.
3. Open the side dampers and sear slide.

4. Set the temperature to 375 degrees F.
5. Smoke the beef for 1 hour and 30 minutes.
6. Flip the beef and smoke for another 1 hour and 30 minutes.
7. Add a Dutch oven on top of the grill.
8. Pour in the olive oil.
9. Add the carrots and potatoes.
10. Cook for 5 minutes.
11. Stir in the garlic and cook for 1 minute.
12. Transfer the beef to the Dutch oven.
13. Stir in the tomato paste, tomato sauce, bell peppers, and water.
14. Bring to a boil.
15. Reduce temperature to 275 degrees F.
16. Simmer for 1 hour.
17. Add the cheese and liver.
18. Season with the salt.

Nutrition Info: Calories: 191.1 Fat: 9.3 g Cholesterol: 34 mg Carbohydrates: 15.4 g Fiber: 1.8 g Sugars: 1.3 g Protein: 11.3 g

Roasted Parmesan Cheese Broccoli

Servings: 3 To 4

Cooking Time: 45 Minutes

Ingredients:

- 3cups broccoli, stems trimmed
- 1tbsp lemon juice
- 1tbsp olive oil
- 2garlic cloves, minced
- 1/2 tsp kosher salt
- 1/2 tsp ground black pepper
- 1tsp lemon zest
- 1/8 cup parmesan cheese, grated

Directions:

1. Preheat pellet grill to 375°F.
2. Place broccoli in a resealable bag. Add lemon juice, olive oil, garlic cloves, salt, and pepper. Seal the bag and toss to combine. Let the mixture marinate for 30 minutes.
3. Pour broccoli into a grill basket. Place basket on grill grates to roast. Grill broccoli for 14-18 minutes, flipping broccoli halfway through. Grill until tender yet a little crispy on the outside.

4. Remove broccoli from grill and place on a serving dish—zest with lemon and top with grated parmesan cheese. Serve immediately and enjoy!
Nutrition Info: Calories: 82.6 Fat: 4.6 g Cholesterol: 1.8 mg Carbohydrate: 8.1 g Fiber: 4.6 g Sugar: 0 Protein: 5.5

Smoked Baked Beans

Servings: 12
Cooking Time: 3 Hours
Ingredients:
- 1 medium yellow onion diced
- 3 jalapenos
- 56 oz pork and beans
- 3/4 cup barbeque sauce
- 1/2 cup dark brown sugar
- 1/4 cup apple cider vinegar
- 2 tbsp Dijon mustard
- 2 tbsp molasses

Directions:
1. Preheat the smoker to 250°F. Pour the beans along with all the liquid in a pan. Add brown sugar, barbeque sauce, Dijon mustard, apple cider vinegar, and molasses. Stir. Place the pan on one of the racks. Smoke for 3 hours until thickened. Remove after 3 hours. Serve
Nutrition Info: Calories: 214 Cal Fat: 2 g Carbohydrates: 42 g   Protein: 7 g Fiber: 7 g

Grilled Ratatouille Salad

Servings: 6
Cooking Time: 25 Minutes
Ingredients:
- 1 Whole sweet potatoes
- 1 Whole red onion, diced
- 1 Whole zucchini
- 1 Whole Squash
- 1 Large Tomato, diced
- As Needed vegetable oil
- As Needed salt and pepper

Directions:
1. Preheat grill to high setting with the lid closed for 10-15 minutes.
2. Slice all vegetables to a ¼ inch thickness.

3. Lightly brush each vegetable with oil and season with Traeger's Veggie Shake or salt and pepper.
4. Place sweet potato, onion, zucchini, and squash on grill grate and grill for 20 minutes or until tender, turn halfway through.
5. Add tomato slices to the grill during the last 5 minutes of cooking time.
6. For presentation, alternate vegetables while layering them vertically. Enjoy!

Wood Pellet Bacon Wrapped Jalapeno Poppers

Servings: 6
Cooking Time: 20 Minutes
Ingredients:
- 6 jalapenos, fresh
- 4 oz cream cheese
- 1/2 cup cheddar cheese, shredded
- 1 tbsp vegetable rub
- 12 slices cut bacon

Directions:
1. Preheat the wood pellet smoker and grill to375°F.
2. Slice the jalapenos lengthwise and scrape the seed and membrane. Rinse them with water and set aside.
3. In a mixing bowl, mix cream cheese, cheddar cheese, vegetable rub until well mixed.
4. Fill the jalapeno halves with the mixture then wrap with the bacon pieces.
5. Smoke for 20 minutes or until the bacon crispy.
6. Serve and enjoy.
Nutrition Info: Calories 1830, Total fat 11g, Saturated fat 6g, Total Carbs 5g, Net Carbs 4g, Protein 6g, Sugar 4g, Fiber 1g

Smoked Balsamic Potatoes And Carrots

Servings: 6
Cooking Time: 10 Minutes
Ingredients:
- 2 large carrots, peeled and chopped roughly
- 2 large Yukon Gold potatoes, peeled and wedged
- 5 tablespoons olive oil
- 5 tablespoons balsamic vinegar

- Salt and pepper to taste

Directions:

1. Fire the Grill to 400F. Use desired wood pellets when cooking. Close the lid and preheat for 15 minutes.

2. Place all ingredients in a bowl and toss to coat the vegetables with the seasoning.

3. Place on a baking tray lined with foil.

4. Place on the grill grate and close the lid. Cook for 30 minutes.

Nutrition Info: Calories per serving: 219; Protein: 2.9g; Carbs: 27g; Fat: 11.4g Sugar:4.5 g

Kale Chips

Servings: 6
Cooking Time: 20 Minutes
Ingredients:

- 2 bunches of kale, stems removed
- ½ teaspoon of sea salt
- 4 tablespoons olive oil

Directions:

1. Switch on the grill, fill the grill hopper with apple-flavored wood pellets, power the grill on by using the control panel, select 'smoke' on the temperature dial, or set the temperature to 250 degrees F and let it preheat for a minimum of 15 minutes.

2. Meanwhile, rinse the kale leaves, pat dry, spread the kale on a sheet tray, drizzle with oil, season with salt and toss until well coated.

3. When the grill has preheated, open the lid, place sheet tray on the grill grate, shut the grill and smoke for 20 minutes until crisp.

4. Serve straight away.

Nutrition Info: Calories: 110 Cal ;Fat: 5 g ;Carbs: 15.8 g ;Protein: 5.3 g ;Fiber: 5.6 g

Garlic And Rosemary Potato Wedges

Servings: 4
Cooking Time: 1 Hour 30 Minutes
Ingredients:

- 4-6 large russet potatoes, cut into wedges
- ¼ cup olive oil
- 2garlic cloves, minced

- 2tablespoons rosemary leaves, chopped
- 2teaspoon salt
- 1teaspoon fresh ground black pepper
- 1teaspoon sugar
- 1teaspoon onion powder

Directions:

1. Preheat your smoker to 250 degrees Fahrenheit using maple wood

2. Take a large bowl and add potatoes and olive oil

3. Toss well

4. Take another small bowl and stir garlic, salt, rosemary, pepper, sugar, onion powder

5. Sprinkle the mix on all sides of the potato wedge

6. Transfer the seasoned wedge to your smoker rack and smoke for 1 and a ½ hours

7. Serve and enjoy!

Nutrition Info: Calories: 291 Fats: 10g Carbs: 46g Fiber: 2g

Smoked Deviled Eggs

Servings: 4 To 6
Cooking Time: 50 Minutes
Ingredients:

- 6 large eggs
- 1slice bacon
- 1/4 cup mayonnaise
- 1tsp Dijon mustard
- 1tsp apple cider vinegar
- 1/4 tsp paprika
- Pinch of kosher salt
- 1tbsp chives, chopped

Directions:

1. Preheat pellet grill to 180°F and turn smoke setting on, if applicable.

2. Bring a pot of water to a boil. Add eggs and hard boil eggs for about 12 minutes.

3. Remove eggs from pot and place them into an ice-water bath. Once eggs have cooled completely, peel them and slice in half lengthwise.

4. Place sliced eggs on grill, yolk side up. Smoke for 30 to 45 minutes, depending on how much smoky flavor you want.

5. While eggs smoke, cook bacon until it's crispy.

6. Remove eggs from the grill and allow to cool on a plate.

7. Remove the yolks and place all of them in a small bowl. Place the egg whites on a plate.

8. Mash yolks with a fork and add mayonnaise, mustard, apple cider vinegar, paprika, and salt. Stir until combined.

9. Spoon a scoop of yolk mixture back into each egg white.

10. Sprinkle paprika, chives, and crispy bacon bits to garnish. Serve and enjoy!

Nutrition Info: Calories: 140 Fat: 12 g Cholesterol: 190 mg Carbohydrate: 1 g Fiber: 0 Sugar: 0 Protein: 6 g

Fries With Chipotle Ketchup

Servings: 6
Cooking Time: 10 Minutes
Ingredients:
- 6 Yukon Gold potatoes, scrubbed and cut into thick strips
- 1 tablespoon Beef Rub
- 1 tablespoon extra-virgin olive oil
- 1 teaspoon onion powder
- 1 teaspoon garlic powder
- ½ cup chipotle peppers, chopped
- 1 cup ketchup
- 1 tablespoon sugar
- 1 tablespoon cumin
- 1 tablespoon chili powder
- 1 whole lime
- 2 tablespoons butter

Directions:
1. Place the potatoes in a bowl and stir in the Beef Rub, olive oil, onion powder, and garlic powder. Toss to coat the potatoes with the spices.
2. Fire the Grill to 500F. Use desired wood pellets when cooking. Close the lid and preheat for 15 minutes.
3. Place the potatoes on a baking sheet lined with foil.
4. Place on the grill grate and cook for 10 minutes.
5. Meanwhile, place the rest of the ingredients in a small bowl and mix until well-combined.
6. Serve the fries with the chipotle ketchup sauce.

Nutrition Info: Calories per serving: 387 ;
Protein: 8.6g; Carbs: 79.3g; Fat: 5.6g Sugar: 13.7g

Roasted Root Vegetables

Servings: 6
Cooking Time: 45 Minutes
Ingredients:
- 1 large red onion, peeled
- 1 bunch of red beets, trimmed, peeled
- 1 large yam, peeled
- 1 bunch of golden beets, trimmed, peeled
- 1 large parsnips, peeled
- 1 butternut squash, peeled
- 1 large carrot, peeled
- 6 garlic cloves, peeled
- 3 tablespoons thyme leaves
- Salt as needed
- 1 cinnamon stick
- Ground black pepper as needed
- 3 tablespoons olive oil
- 2 tablespoons honey

Directions:
1. Switch on the grill, fill the grill hopper with hickory flavored wood pellets, power the grill on by using the control panel, select 'smoke' on the temperature dial, or set the temperature to 450 degrees F and let it preheat for a minimum of 15 minutes.
2. Meanwhile, cut all the vegetables into ½-inch pieces, place them in a large bowl, add garlic, thyme, and cinnamon, drizzle with oil and toss until mixed.
3. Take a large cookie sheet, line it with foil, spread with vegetables, and then season with salt and black pepper.
4. When the grill has preheated, open the lid, place prepared cookie sheet on the grill grate, shut the grill and smoke for 45 minutes until tender.
5. When done, transfer vegetables to a dish, drizzle with honey, and then serve.

Nutrition Info: Calories: 164 Cal ;Fat: 4 g ;Carbs: 31.7 g ;Protein: 2.7 g ;Fiber: 6.4 g

Smoked Pumpkin Soup

Servings: 6
Cooking Time: 1 Hour And 33 Minutes
Ingredients:

- 5 pounds pumpkin, seeded and sliced
- 3 tablespoons butter
- 1 onion, diced
- 2 cloves garlic, minced
- 1 tablespoon brown sugar
- 1 teaspoon paprika
- ¼ teaspoon ground cinnamon
- ¼ teaspoon ground nutmeg
- ½ cup apple cider
- 5 cups broth
- ½ cup cream

Directions:

1. Fire the Grill to 180F. Use desired wood pellets when cooking. Close the lid and preheat for 15 minutes.

2. Place the pumpkin on the grill grate and smoke for an hour or until tender. Allow to cool.

3. Melt the butter in a large saucepan over medium heat and sauté the onion and garlic for 3 minutes. Stir in the rest of the ingredients including the smoked pumpkin. Cook for another 30 minutes.

4. Transfer to a blender and pulse until smooth.

Nutrition Info: Calories per serving: 246; Protein: 8.8g; Carbs: 32.2g; Fat: 11.4g Sugar: 15.5g

Wood Pellet Smoked Vegetables

Servings: 6

Cooking Time: 15 Minutes

Ingredients:

- 1 ear corn, fresh, husks and silk strands removed
- 1yellow squash, sliced
- 1 red onion, cut into wedges
- 1 green pepper, cut into strips
- 1 red pepper, cut into strips
- 1 yellow pepper, cut into strips
- 1 cup mushrooms, halved
- 2 tbsp oil
- 2 tbsp chicken seasoning

Directions:

1. Soak the pecan wood pellets in water for an hour. Remove the pellets from water and fill the smoker box with the wet pellets.

2. Place the smoker box under the grill and close the lid. Heat the grill on high heat for 10 minutes or until smoke starts coming out from the wood chips.

3. Meanwhile, toss the veggies in oil and seasonings then transfer them into a grill basket.

4. Grill for 10 minutes while turning occasionally. Serve and enjoy.

Nutrition Info: Calories 97, Total fat 5g, Saturated fat 2g, Total Carbs 11g, Net Carbs 8g, Protein 2g, Sugar 1g, Fiber 3g, Sodium: 251mg, Potassium 171mg

Grilled Corn On The Cob With Parmesan And Garlic

Servings: 6

Cooking Time: 30 Minutes

Ingredients:

- 4 tablespoons butter, melted
- 2 cloves of garlic, minced
- Salt and pepper to taste
- 8 corns, unhusked
- ½ cup parmesan cheese, grated
- 1 tablespoon parsley chopped

Directions:

1. Fire the Grill to 450F. Use desired wood pellets when cooking. Close the lid and preheat for 15 minutes.

2. Place butter, garlic, salt, and pepper in a bowl and mix until well combined.

3. Peel the corn husk but do not detach the husk from the corn. Remove the silk. Brush the corn with the garlic butter mixture and close the husks.

4. Place the corn on the grill grate and cook for 30 minutes turning the corn every 5 minutes for even cooking.

Nutrition Info: Calories per serving: 272; Protein: 8.8g; Carbs: 38.5g; Fat: 12.3g Sugar: 6.6g

Sweet Potato Chips

Servings: 3

Cooking Time: 35 To 45 Minutes

Ingredients:

- 2 sweet potatoes
- 1 quart warm water

- 1 tablespoon cornstarch, plus 2 teaspoons
- ¼ cup extra-virgin olive oil
- 1 tablespoon salt
- 1 tablespoon packed brown sugar
- 1 teaspoon ground cinnamon
- 1 teaspoon freshly ground black pepper
- ½ teaspoon cayenne pepper

Directions:

1. Using a mandolin, thinly slice the sweet potatoes.
2. Pour the warm water into a large bowl and add 1 tablespoon of cornstarch and the potato slices. Let soak for 15 to 20 minutes.
3. Supply your smoker with wood pellets and follow the manufacturer's specific start-up procedure. Preheat, with the lid closed, to 375°F.
4. Drain the potato slices, then arrange in a single layer on a perforated pizza pan or a baking sheet lined with aluminum foil. Brush the potato slices on both sides with the olive oil.
5. In a small bowl, whisk together the salt, brown sugar, cinnamon, black pepper, cayenne pepper, and the remaining 2 teaspoons of cornstarch. Sprinkle this seasoning blend on both sides of the potatoes.
6. Place the pan or baking sheet on the grill grate, close the lid, and smoke for 35 to 45 minutes, flipping after 20 minutes, until the chips curl up and become crispy.
7. Store in an airtight container.

Roasted Butternut Squash

Servings: 4
Cooking Time: 30 Minutes
Ingredients:

- 2-pound butternut squash
- 3 tablespoon extra-virgin olive oil
- Veggie Rub, as needed

Directions:

1. Fire the Grill to 350F. Use desired wood pellets when cooking. Close the lid and preheat for 15 minutes.
2. Slice the butternut squash into ½ inch thick and remove the seeds. Season with oil and veggie rub.
3. Place the seasoned squash in a baking tray.
4. Grill for 30 minutes.

Nutrition Info: Calories per serving: 131; Protein: 1.9g; Carbs: 23.6g; Fat: 4.7g Sugar: 0g

Potato Fries With Chipotle Peppers

Servings: 4
Cooking Time: 30 Minutes
Ingredients:

- 4 potatoes, sliced into strips
- 3 tablespoons olive oil
- Salt and pepper to taste
- 1 cup mayonnaise
- 2 chipotle peppers in adobo sauce
- 2 tablespoons lime juice

Directions:

1. Set the wood pellet grill to high.
2. Preheat it for 15 minutes while the lid is closed.
3. Coat the potato strips with oil.
4. Sprinkle with salt and pepper.
5. Put a baking pan on the grate.
6. Transfer potato strips to the pan.
7. Cook potatoes until crispy.
8. Mix the remaining ingredients.
9. Pulse in a food processor until pureed.
10. Serve potato fries with chipotle dip.
11. Tips: You can also use sweet potatoes instead of potatoes.

Garlic And Herb Smoke Potato

Servings: 6
Cooking Time: 2 Hours
Ingredients:

- 1.5 pounds bag of Gemstone Potatoes
- 1/4 cup Parmesan, fresh grated
- For the Marinade
- 2 tbsp olive oil
- 6 garlic cloves, freshly chopped
- 1/2 tsp dried oregano
- 1/2 tsp dried basil
- 1/2 tsp dried dill
- 1/2 tsp salt
- 1/2 tsp dried Italian seasoning
- 1/4 tsp ground pepper

Directions:

1. Preheat the smoker to 225°F.

2. Wash the potatoes thoroughly and add them to a sealable plastic bag.

3. Add garlic cloves, basil, salt, Italian seasoning, dill, oregano, and olive oil to the zip lock bag. Shake.

4. Place in the fridge for 2 hours to marinate.

5. Next, take an Aluminum foil and put 2 tbsp of water along with the coated potatoes. Fold the foil so that the potatoes are sealed in

6. Place in the preheated smoker.

7. Smoke for 2 hours

8. Remove the foil and pour the potatoes into a bowl.

9. Serve with grated Parmesan cheese.

Nutrition Info: Calories: 146 Cal Fat: 6 g Carbohydrates: 19 g Protein: 4 g Fiber: 2.1 g

Grilled Zucchini Squash

Servings: 6

Cooking Time: 10 Minutes

Ingredients:

- 3 medium zucchinis, sliced into ¼ inch thick lengthwise
- 2 tablespoons olive oil
- 1 tablespoon sherry vinegar
- 2 thyme leaves, pulled
- Salt and pepper to taste

Directions:

1. Fire the Grill to 350F. Use desired wood pellets when cooking. Close the lid and preheat for 15 minutes.

2. Place zucchini in a bowl and all ingredients. Gently massage the zucchini slices to coat with the seasoning.

3. Place the zucchini on the grill grate and cook for 5 minutes on each side.

Nutrition Info: Calories per serving: 44; Protein: 0.3 g; Carbs: 0.9 g; Fat: 4g Sugar: 0.1g

Minestrone Soup

Servings: 4

Cooking Time: 35 Minutes

Ingredients:

- 1/4 tsp. Black Pepper
- 2tbsp. Olive Oil

- 15 oz. Cannellini Beans
- 1Onion quartered
- 1/2 tsp. Salt
- 2Garlic cloves, minced
- 1/3 cup Parmesan Cheese, grated
- 2Rosemary sprigs, minced
- 1cup Kale leaves, chopped
- 4cups Vegetable Stock
- Juice and Zest of 1 Lemon

Directions:

1. Begin by keeping oil, onion, and garlic in the pitcher of the blender.

2. Next, select the 'saute' button.

3. Once sautéed, stir in celery, rosemary, vegetable stock, lemon zest, lemon juice, kale, parmesan, salt, and pepper.

4. Then, press the 'hearty soup' button.

5. When it takes only 5 to 6 minutes to finish, add the beans and continue cooking.

Nutrition Info: Calories: 34 Fat: 1 g Total Carbs: 4.7 g Fiber: 0.4 g Sugar: 0 g Protein: 1.8 g Cholesterol: 1 mg

Baked Parmesan Mushrooms

Servings: 8

Cooking Time: 15 Minutes

Ingredients:

- 8 mushroom caps
- 1/2 cup Parmesan cheese, grated
- 1/2 teaspoon garlic salt
- 1/4 cup mayonnaise
- Pinch paprika
- Hot sauce

Directions:

1. Place mushroom caps in a baking pan.

2. Mix the remaining ingredients in a bowl.

3. Scoop the mixture onto the mushroom.

4. Place the baking pan on the grill.

5. Cook in the wood pellet grill at 350 degrees F for 15 minutes while the lid is closed.

6. Tips: You can also add chopped sausage to the mixture.

Grilled Zucchini Squash Spears

Servings: 4
Cooking Time: 10 Minutes
Ingredients:
- 4 zucchini, medium
- 2 tbsp olive oil
- 1 tbsp sherry vinegar
- 2 thyme, leaves pulled
- Salt to taste
- Pepper to taste

Directions:
1. Clean zucchini, cut ends off, half each lengthwise, and cut each half into thirds.
2. Combine all the other ingredients in a zip lock bag, medium, then add spears.
3. Toss well and mix to coat the zucchini.
4. Preheat to 350F with the lid closed for about 15 minutes.
5. Remove spears from the zip lock bag and place them directly on your grill grate with the cut side down.
6. Cook for about 3-4 minutes until zucchini is tender and grill marks show.
7. Remove them from the grill and enjoy.

Nutrition Info: Calories 93, Total fat 7.4g, Saturated fat 1.1g, Total carbs 7.1g, Net carbs 4.9g, Protein 2.4g, Sugars 3.4g, Fiber 2.2g, Sodium 59mg, Potassium 515mg

Roasted Veggies & Hummus

Servings: 4
Cooking Time: 20 Minutes
Ingredients:
- 1 white onion, sliced into wedges
- 2 cups butternut squash
- 2 cups cauliflower, sliced into florets
- 1 cup mushroom buttons
- Olive oil
- Salt and pepper to taste
- Hummus

Directions:
1. Set the wood pellet grill to high.
2. Preheat it for 10 minutes while the lid is closed.
3. Add the veggies to a baking pan.
4. Roast for 20 minutes.
5. Serve roasted veggies with hummus.
6. Tips: You can also spread a little hummus on the vegetables before roasting.

Smoked Potato Salad

Servings: 4
Cooking Time: 40 Minutes
Ingredients:
- 2 lb. potatoes
- 2 tablespoons olive oil
- 2 cups mayonnaise
- 1 tablespoon white wine vinegar
- 1 tablespoon dry mustard
- 1/2 onion, chopped
- 2 celery stalks, chopped
- Salt and pepper to taste

Directions:
1. Coat the potatoes with oil.
2. Smoke the potatoes in the wood pellet grill at 180 degrees F for 20 minutes.
3. Increase temperature to 450 degrees F and cook for 20 more minutes.
4. Transfer to a bowl and let cool.
5. Peel potatoes.
6. Slice into cubes.
7. Refrigerate for 30 minutes.
8. Stir in the rest of the ingredients.
9. Tips: You can also add chopped hard-boiled eggs to the mixture.

Wood Pellet Smoked Acorn Squash

Servings: 6
Cooking Time: 2 Hours
Ingredients:
- 3 tbsp olive oil
- 3 acorn squash, halved and seeded
- 1/4 cup unsalted butter
- 1/4 cup brown sugar
- 1 tbsp cinnamon, ground
- 1 tbsp chili powder
- 1 tbsp nutmeg, ground

Directions:

1. Brush olive oil on the acorn squash cut sides then cover the halves with foil. Poke holes on the foil to allow steam and smoke through.
2. Fire up the wood pellet to 225°F and smoke the squash for 1-1/2-2 hours.
3. Remove the squash from the smoker and allow it to sit.
4. Meanwhile, melt butter, sugar and spices in a saucepan. Stir well to combine.
5. Remove the foil from the squash and spoon the butter mixture in each squash half. Enjoy.

Nutrition Info: Calories 149, Total fat 10g, Saturated fat 5g, Total Carbs 14g, Net Carbs 12g, Protein 2g, Sugar 0g, Fiber 2g, Sodium: 19mg, Potassium 0mg

Mexican Street Corn With Chipotle Butter 2

Servings: 6
Cooking Time: 45 Minutes
Ingredients:
- 16 to 20 long toothpicks
- 1 pound Brussels sprouts, trimmed and wilted, leaves removed
- ½ pound bacon, cut in half
- 1 tablespoon packed brown sugar
- 1 tablespoon Cajun seasoning
- ¼ cup balsamic vinegar
- ¼ cup extra-virgin olive oil
- ¼ cup chopped fresh cilantro
- 2 teaspoons minced garlic

Directions:
1. Soak the toothpicks in water for 15 minutes.
2. Supply your smoker with wood pellets and follow the manufacturer's specific start-up procedure. Preheat, with the lid closed, to 300°F.
3. Wrap each Brussels sprout in a half slice of bacon and secure with a toothpick.
4. In a small bowl, combine the brown sugar and Cajun seasoning. Dip each wrapped Brussels sprout in this sweet rub and roll around to coat.
5. Place the sprouts on a Frogmat or parchment paper–lined baking sheet on the grill grate, close the lid, and smoke for 45 minutes to 1 hour, turning as needed, until cooked evenly and the bacon is crisp.

6. In a small bowl, whisk together the balsamic vinegar, olive oil, cilantro, and garlic.
7. Remove the toothpicks from the Brussels sprouts, transfer to a plate and serve drizzled with the cilantro-balsamic sauce.

Roasted Okra

Servings: 4
Cooking Time: 30 Minutes
Ingredients:
- Nonstick cooking spray or butter, for greasing
- 1 pound whole okra
- 2 tablespoons extra-virgin olive oil
- 2 teaspoons seasoned salt
- 2 teaspoons freshly ground black pepper

Directions:
1. Supply your smoker with wood pellets and follow the manufacturer's specific start-up procedure. Preheat, with the lid closed, to 400°F. Alternatively, preheat your oven to 400°F.
2. Line a shallow rimmed baking pan with aluminum foil and coat with cooking spray.
3. Arrange the okra on the pan in a single layer. Drizzle with the olive oil, turning to coat. Season on all sides with the salt and pepper.
4. Place the baking pan on the grill grate, close the lid, and smoke for 30 minutes, or until crisp and slightly charred. Alternatively, roast in the oven for 30 minutes.
5. Serve hot.

Sweet Potato Fries

Servings: 4
Cooking Time: 40 Minutes
Ingredients:
- 3 sweet potatoes, sliced into strips
- 4 tablespoons olive oil
- 2 tablespoons fresh rosemary, chopped
- Salt and pepper to taste

Directions:
1. Set the wood pellet grill to 450 degrees F.
2. Preheat it for 10 minutes.
3. Spread the sweet potato strips in the baking pan.

4. Toss in olive oil and sprinkle with rosemary, salt and pepper.
5. Cook for 15 minutes.
6. Flip and cook for another 15 minutes.
7. Flip and cook for 10 more minutes.
8. Tips: Soak sweet potatoes in water before cooking to prevent browning.

Grilled Cherry Tomato Skewers

Servings: 4
Cooking Time: 50 Minutes
Ingredients:
- 24 cherry tomatoes
- 1/4 cup olive oil
- 3tbsp balsamic vinegar
- 4garlic cloves, minced
- 1tbsp fresh thyme, finely chopped
- 1tsp kosher salt
- 1tsp ground black pepper
- 2tbsp chives, finely chopped

Directions:
1. Preheat pellet grill to 425°F.
2. In a medium-sized bowl, mix olive oil, balsamic vinegar, garlic, and thyme. Add tomatoes and toss to coat.
3. Let tomatoes sit in the marinade at room temperature for about 30 minutes.
4. Remove tomatoes from marinade and thread 4 tomatoes per skewer.
5. Season both sides of each skewer with kosher salt and ground pepper.
6. Place on grill grate and grill for about 3 minutes on each side, or until each side is slightly charred.
7. Remove from grill and allow to rest for about 5 minutes. Garnish with chives, then serve and enjoy!

Nutrition Info: Calories: 228 Fat: 10 g Cholesterol: 70 mg Carbohydrate: 7 g Fiber: 2 g Sugar: 3 g Protein: 27 g

Georgia Sweet Onion Bake

Servings: 6
Cooking Time: 1 Hour
Ingredients:
- Nonstick cooking spray or butter, for greasing

- 4 large Vidalia or other sweet onions
- 8 tablespoons (1 stick) unsalted butter, melted
- 4 chicken bouillon cubes
- 1 cup grated Parmesan cheese

Directions:
1. Supply your smoker with wood pellets and follow the manufacturer's specific start-up procedure. Preheat, with the lid closed, to 350°F.
2. Coat a high-sided baking pan with cooking spray or butter.
3. Peel the onions and cut into quarters, separating into individual petals.
4. Spread the onions out in the prepared pan and pour the melted butter over them.
5. Crush the bouillon cubes and sprinkle over the buttery onion pieces, then top with the cheese.
6. Transfer the pan to the grill, close the lid, and smoke for 30 minutes.
7. Remove the pan from the grill, cover tightly with aluminum foil, and poke several holes all over to vent.
8. Place the pan back on the grill, close the lid, and smoke for an additional 30 to 45 minutes.
9. Uncover the onions, stir, and serve hot.

Salt-crusted Baked Potatoes

Servings: 6
Cooking Time: 40 Minutes
Ingredients:
- 6 russet potatoes, scrubbed and dried
- 3 tablespoons oil
- 1 tablespoons salt
- Butter as needed
- Sour cream as needed

Directions:
1. Fire the Grill to 400F. Use desired wood pellets when cooking. Close the lid and preheat for 15 minutes.
2. In a large bowl, coat the potatoes with oil and salt. Place seasoned potatoes on a baking tray.
3. Place the tray with potatoes on the grill grate.
4. Close the lid and grill for 40 minutes.
5. Serve with butter and sour cream.

Nutrition Info: Calories per serving: 363; Protein: 8g; Carbs: 66.8g; Fat: 8.6g Sugar: 2.3g

Whole Roasted Cauliflower With Garlic Parmesan Butter

Servings: 5
Cooking Time: 45 Minutes
Ingredients:

- 1/4 cup olive oil
- Salt and pepper to taste
- 1 cauliflower, fresh
- 1/2 cup butter, melted
- 1/4 cup parmesan cheese, grated
- 2 garlic cloves, minced
- 1/2 tbsp parsley, chopped

Directions:

1. Preheat the wood pellet grill with the lid closed for 15 minutes.
2. Meanwhile, brush the cauliflower with oil then season with salt and pepper.
3. Place the cauliflower in a cast iron and place it on a grill grate.
4. Cook for 45 minutes or until the cauliflower is golden brown and tender.
5. Meanwhile, mix butter, cheese, garlic, and parsley in a mixing bowl.
6. In the last 20 minutes of cooking, add the butter mixture.
7. Remove the cauliflower from the grill and top with more cheese and parsley if you desire. Enjoy.

Nutrition Info: Calories 156, Total fat 11.1g, Saturated fat 3.4g, Total Carbs 8.8g, Net Carbs 5.1g, Protein 8.2g, Sugar 0g, Fiber 3.7g, Sodium: 316mg, Potassium 468.2mg

Bacon-wrapped Jalapeño Poppers

Servings: 8 To 12
Cooking Time: 40 Minutes
Ingredients:

- 12 large jalapeño peppers
- 8 oz cream cheese, softened
- 1cup pepper jack cheese, shredded
- Juice of 1 lemon1/2 tsp garlic powder
- 1/4 tsp kosher salt
- 1/4 tsp ground black pepper
- 12 bacon slices, cut in half

Directions:

1. Preheat pellet grill to 400°F.

2. Slice jalapeños in half lengthwise. Remove seeds and scrape sides with a spoon to remove the membrane.
3. In a medium bowl, mix cream cheese, pepper jack cheese, garlic powder, salt, and pepper until thoroughly combined.
4. Use a spoon or knife to place the cream cheese mixture into each jalapeño half. Make sure not to fill over the sides of the jalapeño half.
5. Wrap each cheese-filled pepper with a half slice of bacon. If you can't get a secure wrap, then hold bacon and pepper together with a toothpick.
6. Place assembled poppers on the grill and cook for 15-20 minutes or until bacon is crispy.
7. Remove from grill, allow to cool, then serve and enjoy!

Nutrition Info: Calories: 78.8 Fat: 7.2 g Cholesterol: 19.2 mg Carbohydrate: 1 g Fiber: 0.2 g Sugar: 0.7 g Protein: 2.5 g

Roasted Spicy Tomatoes

Servings: 4
Cooking Time: 1 Hour And 30 Minutes
Ingredients:

- 2 lb. large tomatoes, sliced in half
- Olive oil
- 2 tablespoons garlic, chopped
- 3 tablespoons parsley, chopped
- Salt and pepper to taste
- Hot pepper sauce

Directions:

1. Set the temperature to 400 degrees F.
2. Preheat it for 15 minutes while the lid is closed.
3. Add tomatoes to a baking pan.
4. Drizzle with oil and sprinkle with garlic, parsley, salt and pepper.
5. Roast for 1 hour and 30 minutes.
6. Drizzle with hot pepper sauce and serve.
7. Tips: You can also puree the roasted tomatoes and use as sauce for pasta or as dip for chips.

Shiitake Smoked Mushrooms

Servings: 4-6
Cooking Time: 45 Minutes

Ingredients:

- 4 Cup Shiitake Mushrooms
- 1 tbsp canola oil
- 1 tsp onion powder
- 1 tsp granulated garlic
- 1 tsp salt
- 1 tsp pepper

Directions:

1. Combine all the ingredients together
2. Apply the mix over the mushrooms generously.
3. Preheat the smoker at 180°F. Add wood chips and half a bowl of water in the side tray.
4. Place it in the smoker and smoke for 45 minutes.
5. Serve warm and enjoy.

Nutrition Info: Calories: 301 Cal Fat: 9 g Carbohydrates: 47.8 g   Protein: 7.1 g Fiber: 4.8 g

Smoked Eggs

Servings: 12
Cooking Time: 30 Minutes
Ingredients:

- 12 hardboiled eggs, peeled and rinsed

Directions:

1. Supply your smoker with wood pellets and follow the manufacturer's specific start-up procedure. Preheat the grill, with the lid closed, to 120°F.
2. Place the eggs directly on the grill grate and smoke for 30 minutes. They will begin to take on a slight brown sheen.
3. Remove the eggs and refrigerate for at least 30 minutes before serving. Refrigerate any leftovers in an airtight container for 1 or 2 weeks.

Coconut Bacon

Servings: 2
Cooking Time: 30 Minutes
Ingredients:

- 3 1/2 cups flaked coconut
- 1 tbsp pure maple syrup
- 1 tbsp water
- 2 tbsp liquid smoke
- 1 tbsp soy sauce
- 1 tsp smoked paprika (optional)

Directions:

1. Preheat the smoker at 325°F.
2. Take a large mixing bowl and combine liquid smoke, maple syrup, soy sauce, and water.
3. Pour flaked coconut over the mixture. Add it to a cooking sheet.
4. Place in the middle rack of the smoker.
5. Smoke it for 30 minutes and every 7-8 minutes, keep flipping the sides.
6. Serve and enjoy.

Nutrition Info: Calories: 1244 Cal Fat: 100 g Carbohydrates: 70 g   Protein: 16 g Fiber: 2 g

Grilled Broccoli

Servings: 1-2
Cooking Time: 3 Minutes
Ingredients:

- 2cups of broccoli, fresh
- 1tablespoon of canola oil
- 1teaspoon of lemon pepper

Directions:

1. Place the grill; grate inside the unit and close the hood.
2. Preheat the grill by turning at high for 10 minutes.
3. Meanwhile, mix broccoli with lemon pepper and canola oil.
4. Toss well to coat the Ingredients: thoroughly.
5. Place it on a grill grade once add food appears.
6. Lock the unit and cook for 3 minutes at medium.
7. Take out and serve.

Nutrition Info: Calories: 96 Total Fat: 7.3g Saturated Fat: 0.5g Cholesterol: 0mg Sodium: 30mg Total Carbohydrate: 6.7g Dietary Fiber 2.7g Total Sugars: 1.6g Protein: 2.7g

Smoked Baked Kale Chips

Servings: 4
Cooking Time: 30 Minutes
Ingredients:

- 2 bunches kale, stems removed
- Olive oil as needed
- Salt and pepper to taste

Directions:

1. Fire the Grill to 350F. Use desired wood pellets when cooking. Close the lid and preheat for 15 minutes.
2. Place all ingredients in a bowl and toss to coat the kale with oil.
3. Place on a baking tray and spread the leaves evenly on all surface.
4. Place in the grill and cook for 30 minutes or until the kale leaves become crispy.

Nutrition Info: Calories per serving: 206 ;
Protein: 9.9g; Carbs: 21g; Fat: 12g Sugar: 0g

Smokey Roasted Cauliflower

Servings: 4 To 6
Cooking Time: 1 Hour 20 Minutes
Ingredients:
- 1head cauliflower
- cup parmesan cheese
- Spice Ingredients:
- 1tbsp olive oil
- 2cloves garlic, chopped
- 1tsp kosher salt
- 1tsp smoked paprika

Directions:
1. Preheat pellet grill to 180°F. If applicable, set smoke setting to high.
2. Cut cauliflower into bite-size flowerets and place in a grill basket. Place basket on the grill grate and smoke for an hour.
3. Mix spice Ingredients In a small bowl while the cauliflower is smoking. Remove cauliflower from the grill after an hour and let cool.
4. Change grill temperature to 425°F. After the cauliflower has cooled, put cauliflower in a resealable bag, and pour marinade in the bag. Toss to combine in the bag.
5. Place cauliflower back in a grill basket and return to grill. Roast in the grill basket for 10-12 minutes or until the outsides begin to get crispy and golden brown.
6. Remove from grill and transfer to a serving dish. Sprinkle parmesan cheese over the cauliflower and rest for a few minutes so the cheese can melt. Serve and enjoy!

Nutrition Info: Calories: 70 Fat: 35 g Cholesterol: 0 Carbohydrate: 7 g Fiber: 3 g Sugar: 3 g Protein: 3 g

Baked Sweet And Savory Yams

Servings: 6
Cooking Time: 55 Minutes
Ingredients:
- 3 pounds yams, scrubbed
- 3 tablespoons extra virgin olive oil
- Honey to taste
- Goat cheese as needed
- ½ cup brown sugar
- ½ cup pecans, chopped

Directions:
1. Fire the Grill to 350F. Use desired wood pellets when cooking. Close the lid and preheat for 15 minutes.
2. Poke holes on the yams using a fork. Wrap yams in foil and place on the grill grate. Cook for 45 minutes until tender.
3. Remove the yams from the grill and allow to cool. Once cooled, peel the yam and slice to ¼" rounds.
4. Place on a parchment-lined baking tray and brush with olive oil. Drizzle with honey, cheese, brown sugar, and pecans.
5. Place in the grill and cook for another 10 minutes.

Nutrition Info: Calories per serving: 421;
Protein: 4.3g; Carbs: 82.4g; Fat: 9.3g Sugar:19.3 g

Smoked Mushrooms

Servings: 6
Cooking Time: 10 Minutes
Ingredients:
- 4 cups baby portobello, whole and cleaned
- 1 tablespoon canola oil
- 1 teaspoon onion powder
- 1 teaspoon garlic powder
- Salt and pepper to taste

Directions:
1. Place all ingredients in a bowl and toss to coat the mushrooms with the seasoning.

2. Fire the Grill to 350F. Use desired wood pellets when cooking. Close the lid and preheat for 15 minutes.

3. Place mushrooms on the grill grate and smoke for 10 minutes. Make sure to flip the mushrooms halfway through the cooking time.

4. Remove from the grill and serve.

Nutrition Info: Calories per serving: 62; Protein: 5.2g; Carbs: 6.6g; Fat: 2.9g Sugar: 0.3g

Smoked And Smashed New Potatoes

Servings: 4
Cooking Time: 8 Hours
Ingredients:

- 1-1/2 pounds small new red potatoes or fingerlings
- Extra virgin olive oil
- Sea salt and black pepper
- 2 tbsp softened butter

Directions:

1. Let the potatoes dry. Once dried, put in a pan and coat with salt, pepper, and extra virgin olive oil.

2. Place the potatoes on the topmost rack of the smoker.

3. Smoke for 60 minutes.

4. Once done, take them out and smash each one

5. Mix with butter and season

Nutrition Info: Calories: 258 Cal Fat: 2.0 g Carbohydrates: 15.5 g Protein: 4.1 g Fiber: 1.5 g

Butter Braised Green Beans

Servings: 6
Cooking Time: 20 Minutes
Ingredients:

- 24 ounces Green Beans, trimmed
- 8 tablespoons butter, melted
- Salt and pepper to taste

Directions:

1. Fire the Grill to 500F. Use desired wood pellets when cooking. Close the lid and preheat for 15 minutes.

2. Place all ingredients in a bowl and toss to coat the beans with the seasoning.

3. Place the seasoned beans in a sheet tray.

4. Cook in the grill for 20 minutes.

Nutrition Info: Calories per serving: 164; Protein: 1.6g; Carbs: 5.6 g; Fat: 15.8g Sugar: 1.3g

Stuffed Grilled Zucchini

Servings: 4
Cooking Time: 10 Minutes
Ingredients:

- 4 zucchini, medium
- 5 tbsp olive oil, divided
- 2 tbsp red onion, finely chopped
- 1/4 tbsp garlic, minced
- 1/2 cup bread crumbs, dry
- 1/2 cup shredded mozzarella cheese, part-skim
- 1/2 tbsp salt
- 1 tbsp fresh mint, minced
- 3 tbsp parmesan cheese, grated

Directions:

1. Halve zucchini lengthwise and scoop pulp ou. Leave 1/4 -inch shell. Now brush using 2 tbsp oil, set aside, and chop the pulp.

2. Saute onion and pulp in a skillet, large, then add garlic and cook for about 1 minute.

3. Add bread crumbs and cook while stirring for about 2 minutes until golden brown.

4. Remove everything from heat then stir in mozzarella cheese, salt, and mint. Scoop into the zucchini shells and splash with parmesan cheese.

5. Preheat your to 375F.

6. Place stuffed zucchini on the grill and grill while covered for about 8-10 minutes until tender.

7. Serve warm and enjoy.

Nutrition Info: Calories 186, Total fat 10g, Saturated fat 3g, Total carbs 17g, Net carbs 14g, Protein 9g, Sugars 4g, Fiber 3g, Sodium 553mg, Potassium 237mg

Grilled Asparagus & Honey-glazed Carrots

Servings: 4
Cooking Time: 35 Minutes
Ingredients:

- 1 bunch asparagus, woody ends removed
- 2 tbsp olive oil
- 1 lb peeled carrots

- 2 tbsp honey
- Sea salt to taste
- Lemon zest to taste

Directions:

1. Rinse the vegetables under cold water.
2. Splash the asparagus with oil and generously with a splash of salt.
3. Drizzle carrots generously with honey and splash lightly with salt.
4. Preheat your to 350F with the lid closed for about 15 minutes.
5. Place the carrots first on the grill and cook for about 10-15 minutes.
6. Now place asparagus on the grill and cook both for about 15-20 minutes or until done to your liking.
7. Top with lemon zest and enjoy.

Nutrition Info: Calories 184, Total fat 7.3g, Saturated fat 1.1g, Total carbs 28.6g, Net carbs 21g, Protein 6g, Sugars 18.5g, Fiber 7.6g, Sodium 142mg, Potassium 826mg

Roasted Vegetable Medley

Servings: 4 To 6
Cooking Time: 50 Minutes
Ingredients:

- 2medium potatoes, cut to 1 inch wedges
- 2red bell peppers, cut into 1 inch cubes
- 1small butternut squash, peeled and cubed to 1 inch cube
- 1red onion, cut to 1 inch cubes
- 1cup broccoli, trimmed
- 2tbsp olive oil
- 1tbsp balsamic vinegar
- 1tbsp fresh rosemary, minced
- 1tbsp fresh thyme, minced
- 1tsp kosher salt
- 1tsp ground black pepper

Directions:

1. Preheat pellet grill to 425°F.
2. In a large bowl, combine potatoes, peppers, squash, and onion.
3. In a small bowl, whisk together olive oil, balsamic vinegar, rosemary, thyme, salt, and pepper.
4. Pour marinade over vegetables and toss to coat. Allow resting for about 15 minutes.

5. Place marinated vegetables into a grill basket, and place a grill basket on the grill grate. Cook for about 30-40 minutes, occasionally tossing in the grill basket.
6. Remove veggies from grill and transfer to a serving dish. Allow to cool for 5 minutes, then serve and enjoy!

Nutrition Info: Calories: 158.6 Fat: 7.4 g Cholesterol: 0 Carbohydrate: 22 g Fiber: 7.2 g Sugar: 3.1 g Protein: 5.2 g

Corn Chowder

Servings: 3 To 4
Cooking Time: 35 Minutes
Ingredients:

- 1/4 tsp. Cajun Seasoning
- 2tbsp. Butter, unsalted
- 2tbsp. Parsley, fresh and minced
- 1Onion quartered
- 1/2 cup Celery Stalks, diced
- 1/4 tsp. Sea Salt
- 2Garlic cloves
- 1/4 cup Heavy Cream
- 1/2 cup Carrot, diced
- 3cups Corn Kernels, frozen
- 2-1/2 cups Vegetable Broth
- 1/4 tsp. Black Pepper, grounded
- 1Red Potato, chopped

Directions:

1. To start with, keep butter, onion, and garlic in the pitcher of the blender.
2. After that, press the 'saute' button.
3. Next, stir in all the remaining ingredients to the pitcher and select the 'hearty soup' button.
4. Once the program gets over, transfer the soup to serving bowls and serve immediately.
5. Garnish with parsley leaves.

Nutrition Info: Calories: 499 Fat: 40 g Total Carbs: 32 g Fiber: 2.5 g Sugar: 7.3 g Protein: 6.8 g Cholesterol: 120 mg

Carolina Baked Beans

Servings: 12 To 15 Minutes
Cooking Time: 2 To 3 Hours

Ingredients:

- 3 (28-ounce) cans baked beans (I like Bush's brand)
- 1 large onion, finely chopped
- 1 cup The Ultimate BBQ Sauce
- ½ cup light brown sugar
- ¼ cup Worcestershire sauce
- 3 tablespoons yellow mustard
- Nonstick cooking spray or butter, for greasing
- 1 large bell pepper, cut into thin rings
- ½ pound thick-cut bacon, partially cooked and cut into quarters

Directions:

1. Supply your smoker with wood pellets and follow the manufacturer's specific start-up procedure. Preheat, with the lid closed, to 300°F.

2. In a large mixing bowl, stir together the beans, onion, barbecue sauce, brown sugar, Worcestershire sauce, and mustard until well combined

3. Coat a 9-by-13-inch aluminum pan with cooking spray or butter.

4. Pour the beans into the pan and top with the bell pepper rings and bacon pieces, pressing them down slightly into the sauce.

5. Place a layer of heavy-duty foil on the grill grate to catch drips, and place the pan on top of the foil. Close the lid and cook for 2 hours 30 minutes to 3 hours, or until the beans are hot, thick, and bubbly.

6. Let the beans rest for 5 minutes before serving.

POULTRY RECIPES

Glazed Chicken Thighs

Servings: 4
Cooking Time: 30 Minutes
Ingredients:
- 2 garlic cloves, minced
- ¼ C. honey
- 2 tbsp. soy sauce
- ¼ tsp. red pepper flakes, crushed
- 4 (5-oz.) skinless, boneless chicken thighs
- 2 tbsp. olive oil
- 2 tsp. sweet rub
- ¼ tsp. red chili powder
- Freshly ground black pepper, to taste

Directions:
1. Set the temperature of Grill to 400 degrees F and preheat with closed lid for 15 minutes.
2. In a small bowl, add garlic, honey, soy sauce and red pepper flakes and with a wire whisk, beat until well combined.
3. Coat chicken thighs with oil and season with sweet rub, chili powder and black pepper generously.
4. Arrange the chicken drumsticks onto the grill and cook for about 15 minutes per side.
5. In the last 4-5 minutes of cooking, coat the thighs with garlic mixture.
6. Serve immediately.

Nutrition Info: Calories per serving: 309; Carbohydrates: 18.7g; Protein: 32.3g; Fat: 12.1g; Sugar: 17.6g; Sodium: 504mg; Fiber: 0.2g

Authentic Holiday Turkey Breast

Servings: 6
Cooking Time: 4 Hours
Ingredients:
- ½ C. honey
- ¼ C. dry sherry
- 1 tbsp. butter
- 2 tbsp. fresh lemon juice
- Salt, to taste
- 1 (3-3½-pound) skinless, boneless turkey breast

Directions:
1. In a small pan, place honey, sherry and butter over low heat and cook until the mixture becomes smooth, stirring continuously.
2. Remove from heat and stir in lemon juice and salt. Set aside to cool.
3. Transfer the honey mixture and turkey breast in a sealable bag.
4. Seal the bag and shake to coat well.
5. Refrigerate for about 6-10 hours.
6. Set the temperature of Grill to 225-250 degrees F and preheat with closed lid for 15 minutes.
7. Place the turkey breast onto the grill and cook for about 2½-4 hours or until desired doneness.
8. Remove turkey breast from grill and place onto a cutting board for about 15-20 minutes before slicing.
9. With a sharp knife, cut the turkey breast into desired-sized slices and serve.

Nutrition Info: Calories per serving: 443; Carbohydrates: 23.7g; Protein: 59.2g; Fat: 11.4g; Sugar: 23.4g; Sodium: 138mg; Fiber: 0.1g

Lemon Rosemary And Beer Marinated Chicken

Servings: 6
Cooking Time: 55 Minutes
Ingredients:
- 1 whole chicken
- 1 lemon, zested and juiced
- 1 teaspoon salt
- 1 teaspoon ground black pepper
- 1 teaspoon rosemary, chopped
- 12-ounce beer, apple-flavored

Directions:
1. Place all ingredients in a bowl and allow the chicken to marinate for at least 12 hours in the fridge.
2. When ready to cook, fire the Grill to 350F. Use preferred wood pellets. Close the grill lid and preheat for 15 minutes.
3. Place the chicken on the grill grate and cook for 55 minutes.
4. Cook until the internal temperature reads at 165F.

5.	Take the chicken out and allow to rest before carving.
Nutrition Info: Calories per serving: 288; Protein: 36.1g; Carbs: 4.4g; Fat: 13.1g Sugar: 0.7g

Herb Roasted Turkey

Servings: 12
Cooking Time: 3 Hours And 30 Minutes
Ingredients:
- 14 pounds turkey, cleaned
- 2 tablespoons chopped mixed herbs
- Pork and poultry rub as needed
- 1/4 teaspoon ground black pepper
- 3 tablespoons butter, unsalted, melted
- 8 tablespoons butter, unsalted, softened
- 2 cups chicken broth

Directions:
1.	Clean the turkey by removing the giblets, wash it inside out, pat dry with paper towels, then place it on a roasting pan and tuck the turkey wings by tiring with butcher's string.
2.	Switch on the grill, fill the grill hopper with hickory flavored wood pellets, power the grill on by using the control panel, select 'smoke' on the temperature dial, or set the temperature to 325 degrees F and let it preheat for a minimum of 15 minutes.
3.	Meanwhile, prepared herb butter and for this, take a small bowl, place the softened butter in it, add black pepper and mixed herbs and beat until fluffy.
4.	Place some of the prepared herb butter underneath the skin of turkey by using a handle of a wooden spoon, and massage the skin to distribute butter evenly.
5.	Then rub the exterior of the turkey with melted butter, season with pork and poultry rub, and pour the broth in the roasting pan.
6.	When the grill has preheated, open the lid, place roasting pan containing turkey on the grill grate, shut the grill and smoke for 3 hours and 30 minutes until the internal temperature reaches 165 degrees F and the top has turned golden brown.
7.	When done, transfer turkey to a cutting board, let it rest for 30 minutes, then carve it into slices and serve.

Nutrition Info: Calories: 154.6 Cal ;Fat: 3.1 g ;Carbs: 8.4 g ;Protein: 28.8 g ;Fiber: 0.4 g

Lemon Chicken Breast

Servings: 4
Cooking Time: 30 Minutes
Ingredients:
- 6 chicken breasts, skinless and boneless
- ½ cup oil
- 1-3 fresh thyme sprigs
- 1teaspoon ground black pepper
- 2teaspoon salt
- 2teaspoons honey
- 1garlic clove, chopped
- 1lemon, juiced and zested
- Lemon wedges

Directions:
1.	Take a bowl and prepare the marinade by mixing thyme, pepper, salt, honey, garlic, lemon zest, and juice. Mix well until dissolved
2.	Add oil and whisk
3.	Clean breasts and pat them dry, place in a bag alongside marinade and let them sit in the fridge for 4 hours
4.	Preheat your smoker to 400 degrees F
5.	Drain chicken and smoke until the internal temperature reaches 165 degrees, for about 15 minutes
6.	Serve and enjoy!

Nutrition Info: Calories: 230 Fats: 7g Carbs: 1g Fiber: 2g

Peach And Basil Grilled Chicken

Servings: 4
Cooking Time: 35 Minutes
Ingredients:
- 4 boneless chicken breasts
- ½ cup peach preserves, unsweetened
- ½ cup olive oil
- ¼ cup apple cider vinegar
- 3 tablespoons lemon juice
- 2 tablespoons Dijon mustard
- 1 garlic clove, crushed
- ½ teaspoon red hot sauce

- ½ cup fresh basil leaves, chopped
- Salt to taste
- 4 peaches, halved, pit removed

Directions:

1. Place chicken in a bowl and stir in the peach preserves, olive oil, vinegar, lemon juice, Dijon mustard, garlic, red hot sauce, and basil leaves.
2. Massage the chicken until all surfaces are coated with the marinade. Marinate in the fridge for 4 hours.
3. Once ready to cook, fire the Grill to 400F. Use apple wood pellets. Close the lid and preheat for 15 minutes.
4. Place the chicken directly on the grill grate and cook for 35 minutes.
5. Flip the chicken halfway through the cooking time.
6. Ten minutes before the cooking time ends, place the peach halves and grill.
7. Serve with the chicken.

Nutrition Info: Calories per serving: 777; Protein: 61g; Carbs: 9.8g; Fat: 54.2g Sugar: 8g

Beer Can–smoked Chicken

Servings: 3 To 4
Cooking Time: 3 To 4 Hours
Ingredients:

- 8 tablespoons (1 stick) unsalted butter, melted
- ½ cup apple cider vinegar
- ½ cup Cajun seasoning, divided
- 1 teaspoon garlic powder
- 1 teaspoon onion powder
- 1 (4-pound) whole chicken, giblets removed
- Extra-virgin olive oil, for rubbing
- 1 (12-ounce) can beer
- 1 cup apple juice
- ½ cup extra-virgin olive oil

Directions:

1. In a small bowl, whisk together the butter, vinegar, ¼ cup of Cajun seasoning, garlic powder, and onion powder.
2. Use a meat-injecting syringe to inject the liquid into various spots in the chicken. Inject about half of the mixture into the breasts and the other half throughout the rest of the chicken.
3. Rub the chicken all over with olive oil and apply the remaining ¼ cup of Cajun seasoning, being sure to rub under the skin as well.
4. Drink or discard half the beer and place the opened beer can on a stable surface.
5. Place the bird's cavity on top of the can and position the chicken so it will sit up by itself. Prop the legs forward to make the bird more stable, or buy an inexpensive, specially made stand to hold the beer can and chicken in place.
6. Supply your smoker with wood pellets and follow the manufacturer's specific start-up procedure. Preheat, with the lid closed, to 250°F.
7. In a clean 12-ounce spray bottle, combine the apple juice and olive oil. Cover and shake the mop sauce well before each use.
8. Carefully put the chicken on the grill. Close the lid and smoke the chicken for 3 to 4 hours, spraying with the mop sauce every hour, until golden brown and a meat thermometer inserted in the thickest part of the thigh reads 165°F. Keep a piece of aluminum foil handy to loosely cover the chicken if the skin begins to brown too quickly.
9. Let the meat rest for 5 minutes before carving.

Rosemary Orange Chicken

Servings: 6
Cooking Time: 45 Minutes
Ingredients:

- 4 pounds chicken, backbone removed
- For the Marinade:
- 2 teaspoons salt
- 3 tablespoons chopped rosemary leaves
- 2 teaspoons Dijon mustard
- 1 orange, zested
- 1/4 cup olive oil
- ¼ cup of orange juice

Directions:

1. Prepare the chicken and for this, rinse the chicken, pat dry with paper towels and then place in a large baking dish.
2. Prepare the marinade and for this, take a medium bowl, place all of its ingredients in it and whisk until combined.

3. Cover chicken with the prepared marinade, cover with a plastic wrap, and then marinate for a minimum of 2 hours in the refrigerator, turning halfway.

4. When ready to cook, switch on the grill, fill the grill hopper with flavored wood pellets, power the grill on by using the control panel, select 'smoke' on the temperature dial, or set the temperature to 350 degrees F and let it preheat for a minimum of 5 minutes.

5. When the grill has preheated, open the lid, place chicken on the grill grate skin-side down, shut the grill and smoke for 45 minutes until well browned, and the internal temperature reaches 165 degrees F.

6. When done, transfer chicken to a cutting board, let it rest for 10 minutes, cut it into slices, and then serve.

Nutrition Info: Calories: 258 Cal ;Fat: 17.4 g ;Carbs: 5.2 g ;Protein: 19.3 g ;Fiber: 0.3 g

Smo-fried Chicken

Servings: 4 To 6
Cooking Time: 55 Minutes
Ingredients:
- 1 egg, beaten
- ½ cup milk
- 1 cup all-purpose flour
- 2 tablespoons salt
- 1 tablespoon freshly ground black pepper
- 2 teaspoons freshly ground white pepper
- 2 teaspoons cayenne pepper
- 2 teaspoons garlic powder
- 2 teaspoons onion powder
- 1 teaspoon smoked paprika
- 8 tablespoons (1 stick) unsalted butter, melted
- 1 whole chicken, cut up into pieces

Directions:
1. Supply your smoker with wood pellets and follow the manufacturer's specific start-up procedure. Preheat, with the lid closed, to 375°F.
2. In a medium bowl, combine the beaten egg with the milk and set aside.
3. In a separate medium bowl, stir together the flour, salt, black pepper, white pepper, cayenne, garlic powder, onion powder, and smoked paprika.

4. Line the bottom and sides of a high-sided metal baking pan with aluminum foil to ease cleanup.
5. Pour the melted butter into the prepared pan.
6. Dip the chicken pieces one at a time in the egg mixture, and then coat well with the seasoned flour. Transfer to the baking pan.
7. Smoke the chicken in the pan of butter ("smofry") on the grill, with the lid closed, for 25 minutes, then reduce the heat to 325°F and turn the chicken pieces over.
8. Continue smoking with the lid closed for about 30 minutes, or until a meat thermometer inserted in the thickest part of each chicken piece reads 165°F.
9. Serve immediately.

Wood Pellet Smoked Spatchcock Turkey

Servings: 6
Cooking Time: 1 Hour 45 Minutes
Ingredients:
- 1 whole turkey
- 1/2 cup oil
- 1/4 cup chicken rub
- 1 tbsp onion powder
- 1 tbsp garlic powder
- 1 tbsp rubbed sage

Directions:
1. Preheat your wood pellet grill to high.
2. Meanwhile, place the turkey on a platter with the breast side down then cut on either side of the backbone to remove the spine.
3. Flip the turkey and season on both sides then place it on the preheated grill or on a pan if you want to catch the drippings.
4. Grill on high for 30 minutes, reduce the temperature to 325°F, and grill for 45 more minutes or until the internal temperature reaches 165°F
5. Remove from the grill and let rest for 20 minutes before slicing and serving. Enjoy.

Nutrition Info: Calories 156, Total fat 16g, Saturated fat 2g, Total Carbs 1g, Net Carbs 1g, Protein 2g, Sugar 0g, Fiber 0g, Sodium: 19mg

Special Occasion's Dinner Cornish Hen

Servings: 4

Cooking Time: 1 Hour

Ingredients:

- 4 Cornish game hens
- 4 fresh rosemary sprigs
- 4 tbsp. butter, melted
- 4 tsp. chicken rub

Directions:

1. Set the temperature of Grill to 375 degrees F and preheat with closed lid for 15 minutes.
2. With paper towels, pat dry the hens.
3. Tuck the wings behind the backs and with kitchen strings, tie the legs together.
4. Coat the outside of each hen with melted butter and sprinkle with rub evenly.
5. Stuff the cavity of each hen with a rosemary sprig.
6. Place the hens onto the grill and cook for about 50-60 minutes.
7. Remove the hens from grill and place onto a platter for about 10 minutes.
8. Cut each hen into desired-sized pieces and serve.

Nutrition Info: Calories per serving: 430; Carbohydrates: 2.1g; Protein: 25.4g; Fat: 33g; Sugar: 0g; Sodium: 331mg; Fiber: 0.7g

Peppered Bbq Chicken Thighs

Servings: 6
Cooking Time: 35 Minutes

Ingredients:

- 6 bone-in chicken thighs
- Salt and pepper to taste
- Big Game Rub to taste, optional

Directions:

1. Place all ingredients in a bowl and allow to marinate in the fridge for at least 4 hours.
2. When ready to cook, fire the Grill to 350F. Use apple wood pellet. Close the lid and preheat for 15 minutes.
3. Place the chicken directly on the grill grate and cook for 35 minutes. To check if the chicken is cooked thoroughly, insert a meat thermometer, and make sure that the internal temperature reads at 165F.
4. Serve the chicken immediately.

Nutrition Info: Calories per serving: 430; Protein: 32g; Carbs: 1.2g; Fat: 32.1g; Sugar: 0.4g

Jamaican Jerk Chicken Quarters

Servings: 4
Cooking Time: 1 To 2 Hours

Ingredients:

- 4 chicken leg quarters, scored
- ¼ cup canola oil
- ½ cup Jamaican Jerk Paste
- 1 tablespoon whole allspice (pimento) berries

Directions:

1. Supply your smoker with wood pellets and follow the manufacturer's specific start-up procedure. Preheat, with the lid closed, to 275°F.
2. Brush the chicken with canola oil, then brush 6 tablespoons of the Jerk paste on and under the skin. Reserve the remaining 2 tablespoons of paste for basting.
3. Throw the whole allspice berries in with the wood pellets for added smoke flavor.
4. Arrange the chicken on the grill, close the lid, and smoke for 1 hour to 1 hour 30 minutes, or until a meat thermometer inserted in the thickest part of the thigh reads 165°F.
5. Let the meat rest for 5 minutes and baste with the reserved jerk paste prior to serving.

Christmas Dinner Goose

Servings: 12
Cooking Time: 3 Hours

Ingredients:

- 1½ C. kosher salt
- 1 C. brown sugar
- 20 C. water
- 1 (12-lb.) whole goose, giblets removed
- 1 naval orange, cut into 6 wedges
- 1 large onion, cut into 8 wedges
- 2 bay leaves
- ¼ C. juniper berries, crushed
- 12 black peppercorns
- Salt and freshly ground black pepper, to taste
- 1 apple, cut into 6 wedges
- 2-3 fresh parsley sprigs

Directions:

1. Trim off any loose neck skin.
2. Then, trim the first two joints off the wings.
3. Wash the goose under cold running water and with paper towels, pat dry it.
4. With the tip of a paring knife, prick the goose all over the skin.
5. In a large pitcher, dissolve kosher salt and brown sugar in water.
6. Squeeze 3 orange wedges into brine.
7. Add goose, 4 onion wedges, bay leaves, juniper berries and peppercorns in brine and refrigerate for 24 hours.
8. Set the temperature of Grill to 350 degrees F and preheat with closed lid for 15 minutes.
9. Remove the goose from brine and with paper towels, pat dry completely.
10. Season the in and outside of goose with salt and black pepper evenly.
11. Stuff the cavity with apple wedges, herbs, remaining orange and onion wedges.
12. With kitchen strings, tie the legs together loosely.
13. Place the goose onto a rack arranged in a shallow roasting pan.
14. Arrange the goose on grill and cook for about 1 hour.
15. With a basting bulb, remove some of the fat from the pan and cook for about 1 hour.
16. Again, remove excess fat from the pan and cook for about ½-1 hour more.
17. Remove goose from grill and place onto a cutting board for about 20 minutes before carving.
18. With a sharp knife, cut the goose into desired-sized pieces and serve.

Nutrition Info: Calories per serving: 907; Carbohydrates: 23.5g; Protein: 5.6g; Fat: 60.3g; Sugar: 19.9g; Sodium: 8000mg; Fiber: 1.1g

Crispy & Juicy Chicken

Servings: 6
Cooking Time: 5 Hours
Ingredients:

- ¾ C. dark brown sugar
- ½ C. ground espresso beans
- 1 tbsp. ground cumin
- 1 tbsp. ground cinnamon

- 1 tbsp. garlic powder
- 1 tbsp. cayenne pepper
- Salt and freshly ground black pepper, to taste
- 1 (4-lb.) whole chicken, neck and giblets removed

Directions:

1. Set the temperature of Grill to 200-225 degrees F and preheat with closed lid for 15 minutes.
2. In a bowl, mix together brown sugar, ground espresso, spices, salt and black pepper.
3. Rub the chicken with spice mixture generously.
4. Place the chicken onto the grill and cook for about 3-5 hours.
5. Remove chicken from grill and place onto a cutting board for about 10 minutes before carving.
6. With a sharp knife, cut the chicken into desired-sized pieces and serve.

Nutrition Info: Calories per serving: 540; Carbohydrates: 20.7g; Protein: 88.3g; Fat: 9.6g; Sugar: 18.1g; Sodium: 226mg; Fiber: 1.2g

Grill Bbq Chicken Breasts

Servings: 4
Cooking Time: 30 Minutes
Ingredients:

- 4 whole chicken breasts, deboned
- ¼ cup olive oil
- 1 teaspoon pressed garlic
- 1 teaspoon Worcestershire sauce
- 1 teaspoon cayenne pepper powder
- ½ cup 'Que BBQ Sauce

Directions:

1. In a bowl, combine all ingredients except for the 'Que BBQ Sauce and make sure to rub the chicken breasts until coated with the mixture. Allow to marinate in the fridge for at least overnight.
2. Place the preferred wood pellets into the Grill and fire the grill. Allow the temperature to rise to 500F and preheat for 5 minutes. Reduce the temperature to 165F.
3. Place the chicken on the grill grate and cook for 30 minutes.
4. Five minutes before the chicken is done, glaze the chicken with Traeger's BBQ sauce.
5. Serve immediately.

Nutrition Info: Calories per serving: 631; Protein: 61g; Carbs: 2.9g; Fat: 40.5g Sugar: 1.5g

Smoked Turkey Breast

Servings: 2 To 4
Cooking Time: 1 To 2 Hours
Ingredients:
- 1 (3-pound) turkey breast
- Salt
- Freshly ground black pepper
- 1 teaspoon garlic powder

Directions:
1. Supply your smoker with wood pellets and follow the manufacturer's specific start-up procedure. Preheat the grill, with the lid closed, to 180°F.
2. Season the turkey breast all over with salt, pepper, and garlic powder.
3. Place the breast directly on the grill grate and smoke for 1 hour.
4. Increase the grill's temperature to 350°F and continue to cook until the turkey's internal temperature reaches 170°F. Remove the breast from the grill and serve immediately.

Easy Smoked Chicken Breasts

Servings: 4
Cooking Time: 30 Minutes
Ingredients:
- 4 large chicken breasts, bones and skin removed
- 1 tablespoon olive oil
- 2 tablespoons brown sugar
- 2 tablespoons maple syrup
- 1 teaspoon celery seeds
- 2 tablespoons paprika
- 2 tablespoons salt
- 1 teaspoon black pepper
- 2 tablespoons garlic powder
- 2 tablespoons onion powder

Directions:
1. Place all ingredients in a bowl and massage the chicken with your hands. Place in the fridge to marinate for at least 4 hours.

2. Fire the Grill to 350F and use maple wood pellets. Close the lid and allow to preheat to 15 minutes.
3. Place the chicken on the grill a and cook for 15 minutes with the lid closed.
4. Turn the chicken over and cook for another 10 minutes.
5. Insert a thermometer into the thickest part of the chicken and make sure that the temperature reads to 165F.
6. Remove the chicken from the grill and allow to rest for 5 minutes before slicing.
Nutrition Info: Calories per serving: 327 ; Protein: 40 g; Carbs: 23g; Fat: 9g Sugar: 13g

Wood Pellet Sheet Pan Chicken Fajitas

Servings: 10
Cooking Time: 10 Minutes
Ingredients:
- 2 tbsp oil
- 2 tbsp chile margarita seasoning
- 1 tbsp salt
- 1/2 tbsp onion powder
- 1/2 tbsp garlic, granulated
- 2-pound chicken breast, thinly sliced
- 1 red bell pepper, seeded and sliced
- 1 orange bell pepper
- 1 onion, sliced

Directions:
1. Preheat the wood pellet to 450°F. Meanwhile, mix oil and seasoning then toss the chicken and the peppers. Line a sheet pan with foil then place it in the preheated grill. Let it heat for 10 minutes with the grill's lid closed. Open the grill and place the chicken with the veggies on the pan in a single layer. Cook for 10 minutes or until the chicken is cooked and no longer pink. Remove from grill and serve with tortilla or your favorite fixings.
Nutrition Info: Calories: 211 Cal Fat: 6 g Carbohydrates: 5 g   Protein: 29 g Fiber: 1 g

Asian Miso Chicken Wings

Servings: 6
Cooking Time: 25 Minutes

Ingredients:
- 2 lb chicken wings
- 3/4 cup soy
- 1/2 cup pineapple juice
- 1 tbsp sriracha
- 1/8 cup miso
- 1/8 cup gochujang
- 1/2 cup water
- 1/2 cup oil
- Togarashi

Directions:
1. Preheat the to 375F
2. Combine all the ingredients except togarashi in a zip lock bag. Toss until the chicken wings are well coated. Refrigerate for 12 hours
3. Pace the wings on the grill grates and close the lid. Cook for 25 minutes or until the internal temperature reaches 165F
4. Remove the wings from the and sprinkle Togarashi.
5. Serve when hot and enjoy.

Nutrition Info: Calories 703, Total fat 56g, Saturated fat 14g, Total carbs 24g, Net carbs 23g Protein 27g, Sugars 6g, Fiber 1g, Sodium 1156mg

Beer Can Chicken

Servings: 6
Cooking Time: 1 Hour And 15 Minutes
Ingredients:
- 5-pound chicken
- 1/2 cup dry chicken rub
- 1 can beer

Directions:
1. Preheat your wood pellet grill on smoke for 5 minutes with the lid open.
2. The lid must then be closed and then preheated up to 450 degrees Fahrenheit
3. Pour out half of the beer then shove the can in the chicken and use the legs like a tripod.
4. Place the chicken on the grill until the internal temperature reaches 165°F.
5. Remove from the grill and let rest for 20 minutes before serving. Enjoy.

Nutrition Info: Calories: 882 Cal Fat: 51 g
Carbohydrates: 2 g   Protein: 94 g Fiber: 0 g

Roasted Whole Chicken

Servings: 6 To 8
Cooking Time: 1 To 2 Hours
Ingredients:
- 1 whole chicken
- 2 tablespoons olive oil
- 1 batch Chicken Rub

Directions:
1. Supply your smoker with wood pellets and follow the manufacturer's specific start-up procedure. Preheat the grill, with the lid closed, to 375°F.
2. Coat the chicken all over with olive oil and season it with the rub. Using your hands, work the rub into the meat.
3. Place the chicken directly on the grill grate and smoke until its internal temperature reaches 170°F.
4. Remove the chicken from the grill and let it rest for 10 minutes, before carving and serving.

Garlic Parmesan Chicken Wings

Servings: 6
Cooking Time: 20 Minutes
Ingredients:
- 5 pounds of chicken wings
- 1/2 cup chicken rub
- 3 tablespoons chopped parsley
- 1 cup shredded parmesan cheese
- For the Sauce:
- 5 teaspoons minced garlic
- 2 tablespoons chicken rub
- 1 cup butter, unsalted

Directions:
1. Switch on the grill, fill the grill hopper with cherry flavored wood pellets, power the grill on by using the control panel, select 'smoke' on the temperature dial, or set the temperature to 450 degrees F and let it preheat for a minimum of 15 minutes.
2. Meanwhile, take a large bowl, place chicken wings in it, sprinkle with chicken rub and toss until well coated.
3. When the grill has preheated, open the lid, place chicken wings on the grill grate, shut the grill, and

smoke for 10 minutes per side until the internal temperature reaches 165 degrees F.

4. Meanwhile, prepare the sauce and for this, take a medium saucepan, place it over medium heat, add all the ingredients for the sauce in it and cook for 10 minutes until smooth, set aside until required.

5. When done, transfer chicken wings to a dish, top with prepared sauce, toss until mixed, garnish with cheese and parsley and then serve.

Nutrition Info: Calories: 180 Cal ;Fat: 1 g ;Carbs: 8 g ;Protein: 0 g ;Fiber: 0 g

Honey Garlic Chicken Wings

Servings: 4
Cooking Time: 1 Hour And 15 Minutes
Ingredients:
- 2 1/2 lb. chicken wings
- Poultry dry rub
- 4 tablespoons butter
- 3 cloves garlic, minced
- 1/2 cup hot sauce
- 1/4 cup honey

Directions:
1. Sprinkle chicken wings with dry rub.
2. Place on a baking pan.
3. Set the wood pellet grill to 350 degrees F.
4. Preheat for 15 minutes while the lid is closed.
5. Place the baking pan on the grill.
6. Cook for 50 minutes.
7. Add butter to a pan over medium heat.
8. Sauté garlic for 3 minutes.
9. Stir in hot sauce and honey.
10. Cook for 5 minutes while stirring.
11. Coat the chicken wings with the mixture.
12. Grill for 10 more minutes.
13. Tips: You can make the sauce in advance to reduce preparation time.

Wood Pellet Grilled Buffalo Chicken Leg

Servings: 6
Cooking Time: 25 Minutes
Ingredients:
- 12 chicken legs
- 1/2 tbsp salt

- 1 tbsp buffalo seasoning
- 1 cup buffalo sauce

Directions:
1. Preheat your wood pellet grill to 325°F.
2. Toss the legs in salt and buffalo seasoning then place them on the preheated grill.
3. Grill for 40 minutes ensuring you turn them twice through the cooking.
4. Brush the legs with buffalo sauce and cook for an additional 10 minutes or until the internal temperature reaches 165°F.
5. Remove the legs from the grill, brush with more sauce, and serve when hot.

Nutrition Info: Calories: 956 Cal Fat: 47 g Carbohydrates: 1 g Protein: 124 g Fiber: 0 g

Wood Pellet Smoked Spatchcock Turkey

Servings: 6
Cooking Time: 1 Hour And 45 Minutes
Ingredients:
- 1 whole turkey
- 1/2 cup oil
- 1/4 cup chicken rub
- 1 tbsp onion powder
- 1 tbsp garlic powder
- 1 tbsp rubbed sage

Directions:
1. Preheat your wood pellet grill to high.
2. Meanwhile, place the turkey on a platter with the breast side down then cut on either side of the backbone to remove the spine.
3. Flip the turkey and season on both sides then place it on the preheated grill or on a pan if you want to catch the drippings. Grill on high for 30 minutes, reduce the temperature to 325°F, and grill for 45 more minutes or until the internal temperature reaches 165°F Remove from the grill and let rest for 20 minutes before slicing and serving. Enjoy.

Nutrition Info: Calories: 156 Cal Fat: 16 g Carbohydrates: 1 g Protein: 2 g Fiber: 0 g

Chili Barbecue Chicken

Servings: 4
Cooking Time: 2 Hours And 10 Minutes

Ingredients:
- 1 tablespoon brown sugar
- 1 tablespoon lime zest
- 1 tablespoon chili powder
- 1/2 teaspoon ground cumin
- 1/2 tablespoon ground espresso
- Salt to taste
- 2 tablespoons olive oil
- 8 chicken legs
- 1/2 cup barbecue sauce

Directions:
1. Combine sugar, lime zest, chili powder, cumin, ground espresso and salt.
2. Drizzle the chicken legs with oil.
3. Sprinkle sugar mixture all over the chicken.
4. Cover with foil and refrigerate for 5 hours.
5. Set the wood pellet grill to 180 degrees F.
6. Preheat it for 15 minutes while the lid is closed.
7. Smoke the chicken legs for 1 hour.
8. Increase temperature to 350 degrees F.
9. Grill the chicken legs for another 1 hour, flipping once.
10. Brush the chicken with barbecue sauce and grill for another 10 minutes.
11. Tips: You can also add chili powder to the barbecue sauce.

Wood Pellet Grilled Chicken

Servings: 6
Cooking Time: 1 Hour And 10 Minutes
Ingredients:
- 5 pounds whole chicken
- 1/2 cup oil
- Chicken rub

Directions:
1. Preheat your wood pellet on smoke with the lid open for 5 minutes. Close the lid, increase the temperature to 450°F and preheat for 15 more minutes.
2. Tie the chicken legs together with the baker's twine then rub the chicken with oil and coat with chicken rub.
3. Place the chicken on the grill with the breast side up.

4. Grill the chicken for 70 minutes without opening it or until the internal temperature reaches 165°F.
5. Once the chicken is out of the grill let it cool down for 15 minutes
6. Enjoy.
Nutrition Info: Calories: 935 Cal Fat: 53 g Carbohydrates: 0 g   Protein: 107 g Fiber: 0 g

Hickory Smoked Chicken

Servings: 4
Cooking Time: 30 Minutes
Ingredients:
- 4 chicken breasts
- ¼ cup olive oil
- 1 teaspoon pressed garlic
- 1 tablespoon Worcestershire sauce
- Kirkland Sweet Mesquite Seasoning as needed
- 1 button Honey Bourbon Sauce

Directions:
1. Place all ingredients in a bowl except for the Bourbon sauce. Massage the chicken until all parts are coated with the seasoning.
2. Allow to marinate in the fridge for 4 hours.
3. Once ready to cook, fire the Grill to 350F. Use Hickory wood pellets and close the lid. Preheat for 15 minutes.
4. Place the chicken directly into the grill grate and cook for 30 minutes. Flip the chicken halfway through the cooking time.
5. Five minutes before the cooking time ends, brush all surfaces of the chicken with the Honey Bourbon Sauce.
6. Serve immediately.
Nutrition Info: Calories per serving: 622; Protein: 60.5g; Carbs: 1.1g; Fat: 40.3g Sugar: 0.4g

Smoked Turkey Wings

Servings: 2
Cooking Time: 1 Hour
Ingredients:
- 4 turkey wings
- 1 batch Sweet and Spicy Cinnamon Rub

Directions:

1. Supply your smoker with wood pellets and follow the manufacturer's specific start-up procedure. Preheat the grill, with the lid closed, to 180°F.
2. Using your hands, work the rub into the turkey wings, coating them completely.
3. Place the wings directly on the grill grate and cook for 30 minutes.
4. Increase the grill's temperature to 325°F and continue to cook until the turkey's internal temperature reaches 170°F. Remove the wings from the grill and serve immediately.

Wild Turkey Egg Rolls

Servings: 4-6
Cooking Time: 40 Minutes
Ingredients:
- Corn - ½ cup
- Leftover wild turkey meat - 2 cups
- Black beans - ½ cup
- Taco seasoning - 3 tbsp
- Water ½ cup
- Rotel chilies and tomatoes - 1 can
- Egg roll wrappers- 12
- Cloves of minced garlic- 4
- 1 chopped Poblano pepper or 2 jalapeno peppers
- Chopped white onion - ½ cup

Directions:
1. Add some olive oil to a fairly large skillet. Heat it over medium heat on a stove.
2. Add peppers and onions. Sauté the mixture for 2-3 minutes until it turns soft.
3. Add some garlic and sauté for another 30 seconds. Add the Rotel chilies and beans to the mixture. Keeping mixing the content gently. Reduce the heat and then simmer.
4. After about 4-5 minutes, pour in the taco seasoning and ⅓ cup of water over the meat. Mix everything and coat the meat thoroughly. If you feel that it is a bit dry, you can add 2 tbsp of water. Keep cooking until everything is heated all the way through.
5. Remove the content from the heat and box it to store in a refrigerator. Before you stuff the mixture

into the egg wrappers, it should be completely cool to avoid breaking the rolls.
6. Place a spoonful of the cooked mixture in each wrapper and then wrap it securely and tightly. Do the same with all the wrappers.
7. Preheat the pellet grill and brush it with some oil. Cook the egg rolls for 15 minutes on both sides until the exterior is nice and crispy.
8. Remove them from the grill and enjoy with your favorite salsa!
Nutrition Info: Carbohydrates: 26.1 g Protein: 9.2 g Fat: 4.2 g Sodium: 373.4 mg Cholesterol: 19.8 mg

Grilled Buffalo Chicken Legs

Servings: 8
Cooking Time: 1 Hour 15 Minutes;
Ingredients:
- 12 chicken legs
- 1/2 tbsp salt
- 1 tbsp buffalo seasoning
- 1 cup Buffalo sauce

Directions:
1. Preheat your to 325F.
2. Toss the chicken legs in salt and seasoning then place them on the preheated grill.
3. Grill for 40 minutes turning twice through the cooking.
4. Increase the heat and cook for 10 more minutes. Brush the chicken legs and brush with buffalo sauce. Cook for an additional 10 minutes or until the internal temperature reaches 165F.
5. Remove from the and brush with more buffalo sauce.
6. Serve with blue cheese, celery, and hot ranch.
Nutrition Info: Calories 956, Total fat 47g, Saturated fat 13g, Total carbs 1g, Net carbs 1g Protein 124g, Sugars 0g, Fiber 0g, Sodium 1750mg

Wood Pellet Chicken Breasts

Servings: 6
Cooking Time: 15 Minutes
Ingredients:
- 3 chicken breasts
- 1 tbsp avocado oil

- 1/4 tbsp garlic powder
- 1/4 tbsp onion powder
- 3/4 tbsp salt
- 1/4 tbsp pepper

Directions:
1. Preheat your pellet to 375°F.
2. Half the chicken breasts lengthwise then coat with avocado oil.
3. With the spices, drizzle it on all sides to season
4. Drizzle spices to season the chicken. Put the chicken on top of the grill and begin to cook until its internal temperature approaches 165 degrees Fahrenheit. Put the chicken on top of the grill and begin to cook until it rises to a temperature of 165 degrees Fahrenheit
5. Serve and enjoy.

Nutrition Info: Calories: 120 Cal Fat: 4 g Carbohydrates: 0 g   Protein: 19 g Fiber: 0 g

Buttered Thanksgiving Turkey

Servings: 12 To 14
Cooking Time: 5 To 6 Hours
Ingredients:
- 1 whole turkey (make sure the turkey is not pre-brined)
- 2 batches Garlic Butter Injectable
- 3 tablespoons olive oil
- 1 batch Chicken Rub
- 2 tablespoons butter

Directions:
1. Supply your smoker with wood pellets and follow the manufacturer's specific start-up procedure. Preheat the grill, with the lid closed, to 180°F.
2. Inject the turkey throughout with the garlic butter injectable. Coat the turkey with olive oil and season it with the rub. Using your hands, work the rub into the meat and skin.
3. Place the turkey directly on the grill grate and smoke for 3 or 4 hours (for an 8- to 12-pound turkey, cook for 3 hours; for a turkey over 12 pounds, cook for 4 hours), basting it with butter every hour.
4. Increase the grill's temperature to 375°F and continue to cook until the turkey's internal temperature reaches 170°F.

5. Remove the turkey from the grill and let it rest for 10 minutes, before carving and serving.

Buffalo Chicken Wraps

Servings: 4
Cooking Time: 20 Minutes
Ingredients:
- 2 teaspoons poultry seasoning
- 1 teaspoon freshly ground black pepper
- 1 teaspoon garlic powder
- 1 to 1½ pounds chicken tenders
- 4 tablespoons (½ stick) unsalted butter, melted
- ½ cup hot sauce (such as Frank's RedHot)
- 4 (10-inch) flour tortillas
- 1 cup shredded lettuce
- ½ cup diced tomato
- ½ cup diced celery
- ½ cup diced red onion
- ½ cup shredded Cheddar cheese
- ¼ cup blue cheese crumbles
- ¼ cup prepared ranch dressing
- 2 tablespoons sliced pickled jalapeño peppers (optional)

Directions:
1. Supply your smoker with wood pellets and follow the manufacturer's specific start-up procedure. Preheat, with the lid closed, to 350°F.
2. In a small bowl, stir together the poultry seasoning, pepper, and garlic powder to create an all-purpose rub, and season the chicken tenders with it.
3. Arrange the tenders directly on the grill, close the lid, and smoke for 20 minutes, or until a meat thermometer inserted in the thickest part of the meat reads 170°F.
4. In another bowl, stir together the melted butter and hot sauce and coat the smoked chicken with it.
5. To serve, heat the tortillas on the grill for less than a minute on each side and place on a plate.
6. Top each tortilla with some of the lettuce, tomato, celery, red onion, Cheddar cheese, blue cheese crumbles, ranch dressing, and jalapeños (if using).
7. Divide the chicken among the tortillas, close up securely, and serve.

Smoking Duck With Mandarin Glaze

Servings: 4
Cooking Time: 4 Hours
Ingredients:
- 1 quart buttermilk
- 1 (5-pound) whole duck
- ¾ cup soy sauce
- ½ cup hoisin sauce
- ½ cup rice wine vinegar
- 2 tablespoons sesame oil
- 1 tablespoon freshly ground black pepper
- 1 tablespoon minced garlic
- Mandarin Glaze, for drizzling

Directions:
1. With a very sharp knife, remove as much fat from the duck as you can. Refrigerate or freeze the fat for later use.
2. Pour the buttermilk into a large container with a lid and submerge the whole duck in it. Cover and let brine in the refrigerator for 4 to 6 hours.
3. Supply your smoker with wood pellets and follow the manufacturer's specific start-up procedure. Preheat, with the lid closed, to 250°F.
4. Remove the duck from the buttermilk brine, then rinse it and pat dry with paper towels.
5. In a bowl, combine the soy sauce, hoisin sauce, vinegar, sesame oil, pepper, and garlic to form a paste. Reserve ¼ cup for basting.
6. Poke holes in the skin of the duck and rub the remaining paste all over and inside the cavity.
7. Place the duck on the grill breast-side down, close the lid, and smoke for about 4 hours, basting every hour with the reserved paste, until a meat thermometer inserted in the thickest part of the meat reads 165°F. Use aluminum foil to tent the duck in the last 30 minutes or so if it starts to brown too quickly.
8. To finish, drizzle with glaze.

Turkey Meatballs

Servings: 8
Cooking Time: 40 Minutes
Ingredients:
- 1 1/4 lb. ground turkey
- 1/2 cup breadcrumbs
- 1 egg, beaten
- 1/4 cup milk
- 1 teaspoon onion powder
- 1/4 cup Worcestershire sauce
- Pinch garlic salt
- Salt and pepper to taste
- 1 cup cranberry jam
- 1/2 cup orange marmalade
- 1/2 cup chicken broth

Directions:
1. In a large bowl, mix the ground turkey, breadcrumbs, egg, milk, onion powder, Worcestershire sauce, garlic salt, salt and pepper.
2. Form meatballs from the mixture.
3. Preheat the wood pellet grill to 350 degrees F for 15 minutes while the lid is closed.
4. Add the turkey meatballs to a baking pan.
5. Place the baking pan on the grill.
6. Cook for 20 minutes.
7. In a pan over medium heat, simmer the rest of the ingredients for 10 minutes.
8. Add the grilled meatballs to the pan.
9. Coat with the mixture.
10. Cook for 10 minutes.
11. Tips: You can add chili powder to the meatball mixture if you want spicy flavor.

Smoked Lemon Chicken Breasts

Servings: 6
Cooking Time: 30 Minutes
Ingredients:
- 2 lemons, zested and juiced
- 1 clove of garlic, minced
- 2 teaspoons honey
- 2 teaspoons salt
- 1 teaspoon ground black pepper
- 2 sprigs fresh thyme
- ½ cup olive oil
- 6 boneless chicken breasts

Directions:
1. Place all ingredients in a bowl. Massage the chicken breasts so that it is coated with the marinade.
2. Place in the fridge to marinate for at least 4 hours.

3. Fire the Grill to 350F. Use apple wood pellets. Close the grill lid and preheat for 15 minutes.
4. Place the chicken breasts on the grill grate and cook for 15 minutes on both sides.
5. Serve immediately or drizzle with lemon juice.
Nutrition Info: Calories per serving: 671 ; Protein: 60.6 g; Carbs: 3.5 g; Fat: 44.9g Sugar: 2.3g

Smoked Fried Chicken

Servings: 6
Cooking Time: 3 Hours
Ingredients:
- 3.5 lb. chicken
- Vegetable oil
- Salt and pepper to taste
- 2 tablespoons hot sauce
- 1 quart buttermilk
- 2 tablespoons brown sugar
- 1 tablespoon poultry dry rub
- 2 tablespoons onion powder
- 2 tablespoons garlic powder
- 2 1/2 cups all-purpose flour
- Peanut oil

Directions:
1. Set the wood pellet grill to 200 degrees F.
2. Preheat it for 15 minutes while the lid is closed.
3. Drizzle chicken with vegetable oil and sprinkle with salt and pepper.
4. Smoke chicken for 2 hours and 30 minutes.
5. In a bowl, mix the hot sauce, buttermilk and sugar.
6. Soak the smoked chicken in the mixture.
7. Cover and refrigerate for 1 hour.
8. In another bowl, mix the dry rub, onion powder, garlic powder and flour.
9. Coat the chicken with the mixture.
10. Heat the peanut oil in a pan over medium heat.
11. Fry the chicken until golden and crispy.
12. Tips: Drain chicken on paper towels before serving.

Buffalo Chicken Flatbread

Servings: 6
Cooking Time: 30 Minutes

Ingredients:
- 6 mini pita bread
- 1-1/2 cups buffalo sauce
- 4 cups chicken breasts, cooked and cubed
- 3 cups mozzarella cheese
- Blue cheese for drizzling

Directions:
1. Preheat the wood pellet grill to 375-400°F.
2. Place the breads on a flat surface and evenly spread sauce over all of them.
3. Toss the chicken with the remaining buffalo sauce and place it on the pita breads.
4. Top with cheese then place the breads on the grill but indirectly from the heat. Close the grill lid.
5. Cook for 7 minutes or until the cheese has melted and the edges are toasty.
6. Remove from grill and drizzle with blue cheese. Serve and enjoy.
Nutrition Info: Calories: 254 Cal Fat: 13 g Carbohydrates: 4 g   Protein: 33 g Fiber: 3 g

Cinco De Mayo Chicken Enchiladas

Servings: 6
Cooking Time: 45 Minutes
Ingredients:
- 6 cups diced cooked chicken
- 3 cups grated Monterey Jack cheese, divided
- 1 cup sour cream
- 1 (4-ounce) can chopped green chiles
- 2 (10-ounce) cans red or green enchilada sauce, divided
- 12 (8-inch) flour tortillas
- ½ cup chopped scallions
- ¼ cup chopped fresh cilantro

Directions:
1. Supply your smoker with wood pellets and follow the manufacturer's specific start-up procedure. Preheat, with the lid closed, to 350°F.
2. In a large bowl, combine the cooked chicken, 2 cups of cheese, the sour cream, and green chiles to make the filling.
3. Pour one can of enchilada sauce in the bottom of a 9-by-13-inch baking dish or aluminum pan.
4. Spoon ⅓ cup of the filling on each tortilla and roll up securely.

5. Transfer the tortillas seam-side down to the baking dish, then pour the remaining can of enchilada sauce over them, coating all exposed surfaces of the tortillas.

6. Sprinkle the remaining 1 cup of cheese over the enchiladas and cover tightly with aluminum foil.

7. Bake on the grill, with the lid closed, for 30 minutes, then remove the foil.

8. Continue baking with the lid closed for 15 minutes, or until bubbly.

9. Garnish the enchiladas with the chopped scallions and cilantro and serve immediately.

Sweet And Spicy Smoked Wings

Servings: 2 To 4
Cooking Time: 1 Hour, 25 Minutes
Ingredients:
- 1 pound chicken wings
- 1 batch Sweet and Spicy Cinnamon Rub
- 1 cup barbecue sauce

Directions:

1. Supply your smoker with wood pellets and follow the manufacturer's specific start-up procedure. Preheat the grill, with the lid closed, to 325°F.

2. Season the chicken wings with the rub. Using your hands, work the rub into the meat.

3. Place the wings directly on the grill grate and cook until they reach an internal temperature of 165°F.

4. Transfer the wings into an aluminum pan. Add the barbecue sauce and stir to coat the wings.

5. Reduce the grill's temperature to 250°F and put the pan on the grill. Smoke the wings for 1 hour more, uncovered. Remove the wings from the grill and serve immediately.

Cajun Chicken

Servings: 4
Cooking Time: 30 Minutes
Ingredients:
- 2 lb. chicken wings
- Poultry dry rub
- Cajun seasoning

Directions:

1. Season the chicken wings with the dry rub and Cajun seasoning.

2. Preheat the to 350 degrees F for 15 minutes while the lid is closed.

3. Grill for 30 minutes, flipping twice.

4. Tips: You can also smoke the chicken before grilling.

Turkey Breast

Servings: 6
Cooking Time: 8 Hours
Ingredients:
- For the Brine:
- 2 pounds turkey breast, deboned
- 2 tablespoons ground black pepper
- 1/4 cup salt
- 1 cup brown sugar
- 4 cups cold water
- For the BBQ Rub:
- 2 tablespoons dried onions
- 2 tablespoons garlic powder
- 1/4 cup paprika
- 2 tablespoons ground black pepper
- 1 tablespoon salt
- 2 tablespoons brown sugar
- 2 tablespoons red chili powder
- 1 tablespoon cayenne pepper
- 2 tablespoons sugar
- 2 tablespoons ground cumin

Directions:

1. Prepare the brine and for this, take a large bowl, add salt, black pepper, and sugar in it, pour in water, and stir until sugar has dissolved.

2. Place turkey breast in it, submerge it completely and let it soak for a minimum of 12 hours in the refrigerator.

3. Meanwhile, prepare the BBQ rub and for this, take a small bowl, place all of its ingredients in it and then stir until combined, set aside until required.

4. Then remove turkey breast from the brine and season well with the prepared BBQ rub.

5. When ready to cook, switch on the grill, fill the grill hopper with apple-flavored wood pellets, power the grill on by using the control panel, select 'smoke' on the temperature dial, or set the temperature to

180 degrees F and let it preheat for a minimum of 15 minutes.

6. When the grill has preheated, open the lid, place turkey breast on the grill grate, shut the grill, change the smoking temperature to 225 degrees F, and smoke for 8 hours until the internal temperature reaches 160 degrees F.

7. When done, transfer turkey to a cutting board, let it rest for 10 minutes, then cut it into slices and serve.

Nutrition Info: Calories: 250 Cal ;Fat: 5 g ;Carbs: 31 g ;Protein: 18 g ;Fiber: 5 g

Rustic Maple Smoked Chicken Wings

Servings: 16
Cooking Time: 35 Minutes
Ingredients:
- 16 chicken wings
- 1 tablespoon olive oil
- 1 tablespoon Chicken Rub
- 1 cup 'Que BBQ Sauce or other commercial BBQ sauce of choice

Directions:
1. Place all ingredients in a bowl except for the BBQ sauce. Massage the chicken breasts so that it is coated with the marinade.
2. Place in the fridge to marinate for at least 4 hours.
3. Fire the Grill to 350F. Use maple wood pellets. Close the grill lid and preheat for 15 minutes.
4. Place the wings on the grill grate and cook for 12 minutes on each side with the lid closed.
5. Once the chicken wings are done, place in a clean bowl.
6. Pour over the BBQ sauce and toss to coat with the sauce.

Nutrition Info: Calories per serving: 230 ; Protein: 37.5g; Carbs: 2.2g; Fat: 7g Sugar: 1.3g

Sheet Pan Chicken Fajitas

Servings: 10
Cooking Time: 10 Minutes
Ingredients:
- 2 lb chicken breast

- 1 onion, sliced
- 1 red bell pepper, seeded and sliced
- 1 orange-red bell pepper, seeded and sliced
- 1 tbsp salt
- 1/2 tbsp onion powder
- 1/2 tbsp granulated garlic
- 2 tbsp Spiceologist Chile Margarita Seasoning
- 2 tbsp oil

Directions:
1. Preheat the to 450F and line a baking sheet with parchment paper.
2. In a mixing bowl, combine seasonings and oil then toss with the peppers and chicken.
3. Place the baking sheet in the and let heat for 10 minutes with the lid closed.
4. Open the lid and place the veggies and the chicken in a single layer. Close the lid and cook for 10 minutes or until the chicken is no longer pink.
5. Serve with warm tortillas and top with your favorite toppings.

Nutrition Info: Calories 211, Total fat 6g, Saturated fat 1g, Total carbs 5g, Net carbs 4g Protein 29g, Sugars 4g, Fiber 1g, Sodium 360mg

Chinese Inspired Duck Legs

Servings: 8
Cooking Time: 1 Hour 10 Minutes
Ingredients:
- For Glaze:
- ¼ C. fresh orange juice
- ¼ C. orange marmalade
- ¼ C. mirin
- 2 tbsp. hoisin sauce
- ½ tsp. red pepper flakes, crushed
- For Duck:
- 1 tsp. kosher salt
- ¾ tsp. freshly ground black pepper
- ¾ tsp. Chinese five-spice powder
- 8 (6-oz.) duck legs

Directions:
1. Set the temperature of Grill to 235 degrees F and preheat with closed lid for 15 minutes.
2. Forb glaze: in a small pan, add all ingredients over medium-high heat and bring to gentle boil, stirring continuously.

3. Remove from heat and set aside.

4. For rub: in a small bowl, mix together salt, black pepper and five-spice powder.

5. Rub the duck legs with spice rub evenly.

6. Place the duck legs onto the grill, skin side up and cook for about 50 minutes.

7. Coat the duck legs with glaze ad cook for about 20 minutes, flipping and coating with glaze after every 5 minutes.

Nutrition Info: Calories per serving: 303; Carbohydrates: 0.1g; Protein: 49.5g; Fat: 10.2g; Sugar: 0g; Sodium: 474mg; Fiber: 0.1g

Paprika Chicken

Servings: 7
Cooking Time: 2 – 4 Hours
Ingredients:
- 4-6 chicken breast
- 4 tablespoons olive oil
- 2tablespoons smoked paprika
- ½ tablespoon salt
- ¼ teaspoon pepper
- 2teaspoons garlic powder
- 2teaspoons garlic salt
- 2teaspoons pepper
- 1teaspoon cayenne pepper
- 1teaspoon rosemary

Directions:
1. Preheat your smoker to 220 degrees Fahrenheit using your favorite wood Pellets

2. Prepare your chicken breast according to your desired shapes and transfer to a greased baking dish

3. Take a medium bowl and add spices, stir well

4. Press the spice mix over chicken and transfer the chicken to smoker

5. Smoke for 1-1 and a ½ hours

6. Turn-over and cook for 30 minutes more

7. Once the internal temperature reaches 165 degrees Fahrenheit

8. Remove from the smoker and cover with foil

9. Allow it to rest for 15 minutes

10. Enjoy!

Nutrition Info: Calories: 237 Fats: 6.1g Carbs: 14g Fiber: 3g

Grilled Chicken

Servings: 6
Cooking Time: 1 Hour 10 Minutes;
Ingredients:
- 5 lb. whole chicken
- 1/2 cup oil
- chicken rub

Directions:
1. Preheat the on the smoke setting with the lid open for 5 minutes. Close the lid and let it heat for 15 minutes or until it reaches 450..

2. Use bakers twine to tie the chicken legs together then rub it with oil. Coat the chicken with the rub and place it on the grill.

3. Grill for 70 minutes with the lid closed or until it reaches an internal temperature of 165F.

4. Remove the chicken from the and let rest for 15 minutes. Cut and serve.

Nutrition Info: Calories 935, Total fat 53g, Saturated fat 15g, Total carbs 0g, Net carbs 0g Protein 107g, Sugars 0g, Fiber 0g, Sodium 320mg

Perfectly Smoked Turkey Legs

Servings: 6
Cooking Time: 4 Hours
Ingredients:
- For Turkey:
- 3 tbsp. Worcestershire sauce
- 1 tbsp. canola oil
- 6 turkey legs
- For Rub:
- ¼ C. chipotle seasoning
- 1 tbsp. brown sugar
- 1 tbsp. paprika
- For Sauce:
- 1 C. white vinegar
- 1 tbsp. canola oil
- 1 tbsp. chipotle BBQ sauce

Directions:
1. For turkey in a bowl, add the Worcestershire sauce and canola oil and mix well.

2. With your fingers, loosen the skin of legs.

3. With your fingers coat the legs under the skin with oil mixture.

4. In another bowl, mix together rub ingredients.

5. Rub the spice mixture under and outer surface of turkey legs generously.

6. Transfer the legs into a large sealable bag and refrigerate for about 2-4 hours.

7. Remove the turkey legs from refrigerator and set aside at room temperature for at least 30 minutes before cooking.

8. Set the temperature of Grill to 200-220 degrees F and preheat with closed lid for 15 minutes.

9. In a small pan, mix together all sauce ingredients on low heat and cook until warmed completely, stirring continuously.

10. Place the turkey legs onto the grill cook for about 3½-4 hours, coating with sauce after every 45 minutes.

11. Serve hot.

Nutrition Info: Calories per serving: 430; Carbohydrates: 4.9g; Protein: 51.2g; Fat: 19.5g; Sugar: 3.9g; Sodium: 1474mg; Fiber: 0.5g

Chicken Wings

Servings: 4
Cooking Time: 15 Minutes
Ingredients:
- Fresh chicken wings
- Salt to taste
- Pepper to taste
- Garlic powder
- Onion powder
- Cayenne
- Paprika
- Seasoning salt
- Barbeque sauce to taste

Directions:
1. Preheat the wood pellet grill to low. Mix seasoning and coat on chicken. Put the wings on the grill and cook. Place the wings on the grill and cook for 20 minutes or until the wings are fully cooked. Let rest to cool for 5 minutes then toss with barbeque sauce. Serve with orzo and salad. Enjoy.

Nutrition Info: Calories: 311 Cal Fat: 22 g Carbohydrates: 22 g Protein: 22 g Fiber: 3 g

Turkey With Apricot Barbecue Glaze

Servings: 4
Cooking Time: 30 Minutes
Ingredients:
- 4 turkey breast fillets
- 4 tablespoons chicken rub
- 1 cup apricot barbecue sauce

Directions:
1. Preheat the wood pellet grill to 365 degrees F for 15 minutes while the lid is closed.

2. Season the turkey fillets with the chicken run.

3. Grill the turkey fillets for 5 minutes per side.

4. Brush both sides with the barbecue sauce and grill for another 5 minutes per side.

5. Tips: You can sprinkle turkey with chili powder if you want your dish spicy.

Smoked Whole Duck

Servings: 6
Cooking Time: 2 Hours 30 Minutes
Ingredients:
- 5 pounds whole duck (trimmed of any excess fat)
- 1small onion (quartered)
- 1apple (wedged)
- 1orange (quartered)
- 1tbsp freshly chopped parsley
- 1tbsp freshly chopped sage
- ½ tsp onion powder
- 2tsp smoked paprika
- 1tsp dried Italian seasoning
- 1tbsp dried Greek seasoning
- 1tsp pepper or to taste
- 1tsp sea salt or to taste

Directions:
1. Remove giblets and rinse duck, inside and pour, under cold running water.

2. Pat dry with paper towels.

3. Use the tip of a sharp knife to cut the duck skin all over. Be careful not to cut through the meat. Tie the duck legs together with butcher's string.

4. To make a rub, combine the onion powder, pepper, salt, Italian seasoning, Greek seasoning, and paprika in a mixing bowl.

5. Insert the orange, onion, and apple to the duck cavity. Stuff the duck with freshly chopped parsley and sage.

6. Season all sides of the duck generously with rub mixture.

7. Start your pellet grill on smoke mode, leaving the lip open or until the fire starts.

8. Close the lid and preheat the grill to 325°F for 10 minutes.

9. Place the duck on the grill grate.

10. Roast for 2 to 21/2 hours, or until the duck skin is brown and the internal temperature of the thigh reaches 160°F.

11. Remove the duck from heat and let it rest for a few minutes.

12. Cut into sizes and serve.

Nutrition Info: Calories: 809 Total Fat: 42.9 g Saturated Fat: 15.8 g Cholesterol: 337 mg Sodium: 638 mg Total Carbohydrate: 11.7 g Dietary Fiber: 2.4 g Total Sugars: 7.5 g Protein: 89.6 g

Maple And Bacon Chicken

Servings: 7
Cooking Time: 1 And ½ Hours
Ingredients:
- 4 boneless and skinless chicken breast
- Salt as needed
- Fresh pepper
- 12 slices bacon, uncooked
- 1cup maple syrup
- ½ cup melted butter
- 1teaspoon liquid smoke

Directions:
1. Preheat your smoker to 250 degrees Fahrenheit
2. Season the chicken with pepper and salt
3. Wrap the breast with 3 bacon slices and cover the entire surface
4. Secure the bacon with toothpicks
5. Take a medium-sized bowl and stir in maple syrup, butter, liquid smoke, and mix well
6. Reserve 1/3rd of this mixture for later use
7. Submerge the chicken breast into the butter mix and coat them well

8. Place a pan in your smoker and transfer the chicken to your smoker

9. Smoker for 1 to 1 and a ½ hours

10. Brush the chicken with reserved butter and smoke for 30 minutes more until the internal temperature reaches 165 degrees Fahrenheit

11. Enjoy!

Nutrition Info: Calories: 458 Fats: 20g Carbs: 65g Fiber: 1g

Bbq Sauce Smothered Chicken Breasts

Servings: 4
Cooking Time: 30 Minutes
Ingredients:
- 1 tsp. garlic, crushed
- ¼ C. olive oil
- 1 tbsp. Worcestershire sauce
- 1 tbsp. sweet mesquite seasoning
- 4 chicken breasts
- 2 tbsp. regular BBQ sauce
- 2 tbsp. spicy BBQ sauce
- 2 tbsp. honey bourbon BBQ sauce

Directions:
1. Set the temperature of Grill to 450 degrees F and preheat with closed lid for 15 minutes.
2. In a large bowl, mix together garlic, oil, Worcestershire sauce and mesquite seasoning.
3. Coat chicken breasts with seasoning mixture evenly.
4. Place the chicken breasts onto the grill and cook for about 20-30 minutes.
5. Meanwhile, in a bowl, mix together all 3 BBQ sauces.
6. In the last 4-5 minutes of cooking, coat breast with BBQ sauce mixture.
7. Serve hot.

Nutrition Info: Calories per serving: 421; Carbohydrates: 10.1g; Protein: 41,2g; Fat: 23.3g; Sugar: 6.9g; Sodium: 763mg; Fiber: 0.2g

Wood Pellet Smoked Cornish Hens

Servings: 6

Cooking Time: 1 Hour

Ingredients:

- 6 Cornish hens
- 3 tbsp avocado oil
- 6 tbsp rub of choice

Directions:

1. Fire up the wood pellet and preheat it to 275°F.
2. Rub the hens with oil then coat generously with rub. Place the hens on the grill with the chest breast side down.
3. Smoke for 30 minutes. Flip the hens and increase the grill temperature to 400°F. Cook until the internal temperature reaches 165°F.
4. Remove from the grill and let rest for 10 minutes before serving. Enjoy.

Nutrition Info: Calories: 696 Cal Fat: 50 g Carbohydrates: 1 g Protein: 57 g Fiber: 0 g

- Poultry Rub to taste

Directions:

1. Place all ingredients in a bowl and mix until the chicken pieces are coated in oil and rub. Allow to marinate for at least 2 hours.
2. Fire the Grill to 180F. Close the lid and allow to preheat for 10 minutes. Use hickory wood pellets to smoke your chicken.
3. Arrange the chicken on the grill grate and smoke for one hour. Increase the temperature to 350F and continue cooking for another hour until the chicken is golden and the juices run clean.
4. To check if the meat is cooked, insert a meat thermometer, and make sure that the temperature on the thickest part of the chicken registers at 165F.
5. Remove the chicken and serve.

Nutrition Info: Calories per serving: 358 ; Protein: 50.8g; Carbs: 0g; Fat: 15.7g Sugar:0 g

Wood Pellet Chile Lime Chicken

Servings: 1

Cooking Time: 15 Minutes

Ingredients:

- 1 chicken breast
- 1 tbsp oil
- 1 tbsp chile-lime seasoning

Directions:

1. Preheat your wood pellet to 400°F.
2. Brush the chicken breast with oil on all sides.
3. Sprinkle with seasoning and salt to taste.
4. Grill for 7 minutes per side or until the internal temperature reaches 165°F.
5. Serve when hot or cold and enjoy.

Nutrition Info: Calories: 131 Cal Fat: 5 g Carbohydrates: 4 g Protein: 19 g Fiber: 1 g

Hickory Smoked Chicken Leg And Thigh Quarters

Servings: 6

Cooking Time: 2 Hours

Ingredients:

- 6 chicken legs (with thigh and drumsticks)
- 2 tablespoons olive oil

Buffalo Wings

Servings: 2 To 3

Cooking Time: 35 Minutes

Ingredients:

- 1 pound chicken wings
- 1 batch Chicken Rub
- 1 cup Frank's Red-Hot Sauce, Buffalo wing sauce, or similar

Directions:

1. Supply your smoker with wood pellets and follow the manufacturer's specific start-up procedure. Preheat the grill, with the lid closed, to 300°F.
2. Season the chicken wings with the rub. Using your hands, work the rub into the meat.
3. Place the wings directly on the grill grate and smoke until their internal temperature reaches 160°F.
4. Baste the wings with the sauce and continue to smoke until the wings' internal temperature reaches 170°F.

Spatchcocked Turkey

Servings: 10 To 14

Cooking Time: 2 Hours

Ingredients:

- 1 whole turkey
- 2 tablespoons olive oil
- 1 batch Chicken Rub

Directions:

1. Supply your smoker with wood pellets and follow the manufacturer's specific start-up procedure. Preheat the grill, with the lid closed, to 350°F.

2. To remove the turkey's backbone, place the turkey on a work surface, on its breast. Using kitchen shears, cut along one side of the turkey's backbone and then the other. Pull out the bone.

3. Once the backbone is removed, turn the turkey breast-side up and flatten it.

4. Coat the turkey with olive oil and season it on both sides with the rub. Using your hands, work the rub into the meat and skin.

5. Place the turkey directly on the grill grate, breast-side up, and cook until its internal temperature reaches 170°F.

6. Remove the turkey from the grill and let it rest for 10 minutes, before carving and serving.

Wood-fired Chicken Breasts

Servings: 2 To 4

Cooking Time: 45 Minutes

Ingredients:

- 2 (1-pound) bone-in, skin-on chicken breasts
- 1 batch Chicken Rub

Directions:

1. Supply your smoker with wood pellets and follow the manufacturer's specific start-up procedure. Preheat the grill, with the lid closed, to 350°F.

2. Season the chicken breasts all over with the rub. Using your hands, work the rub into the meat.

3. Place the breasts directly on the grill grate and smoke until their internal temperature reaches 170°F. Remove the breasts from the grill and serve immediately.

Hot And Sweet Spatchcocked Chicken

Servings: 8

Cooking Time: 55 Minutes

Ingredients:

- 1 whole chicken, spatchcocked
- ¼ cup Chicken Rub
- 2 tablespoons olive oil
- ½ cup Sweet and Heat BBQ Sauce

Directions:

1. Place the chicken breastbone-side down on a flat surface and press the breastbone to break it and flatten the chicken. Sprinkle the Chicken Rub all over the chicken and massage until the bird is seasoned well. Allow the chicken to rest in the fridge for at least 12 hours.

2. When ready to cook, fire the Grill to 350F. Use preferred wood pellets. Close the grill lid and preheat for 15 minutes.

3. Before cooking the chicken, baste with oil. Place on the grill grate and cook on both sides for 55 minutes.

4. 20 minutes before the cooking time, baste the chicken with Sweet and Heat BBQ Sauce.

5. Continue cooking until a meat thermometer inserted in the thickest part of the chicken reads at 165F.

6. Allow to rest before carving the chicken.

Nutrition Info: Calories per serving: 200; Protein: 30.6g; Carbs: 1.1g; Fat: 7.4g Sugar: 0.6g

Wild West Wings

Servings: 4

Cooking Time: 1 Hour

Ingredients:

- 2 pounds chicken wings
- 2 tablespoons extra-virgin olive oil
- 2 packages ranch dressing mix (such as Hidden Valley brand)
- ¼ cup prepared ranch dressing (optional)

Directions:

1. Supply your smoker with wood pellets and follow the manufacturer's specific start-up procedure. Preheat, with the lid closed, to 350°F.

2. Place the chicken wings in a large bowl and toss with the olive oil and ranch dressing mix.

3. Arrange the wings directly on the grill, or line the grill with aluminum foil for easy cleanup, close the lid, and smoke for 25 minutes.

4. Flip and smoke for 20 to 35 minutes more, or until a meat thermometer inserted in the thickest part of the wings reads 165°F and the wings are crispy. (Note: The wings will likely be done after 45 minutes, but an extra 10 to 15 minutes makes them crispy without drying the meat.)

5. Serve warm with ranch dressing (if using).

BEEF,PORK & LAMB RECIPES

Bbq Sweet Pepper Meatloaf

Servings: 8

Cooking Time: 3 Hours And 15 Minutes

Ingredients:

- 1 cup chopped red sweet peppers
- 5 pounds ground beef
- 1 cup chopped green onion
- 1 tablespoon salt
- 1 tablespoon ground black pepper
- 1 cup panko bread crumbs
- 2 tablespoon BBQ rub and more as needed
- 1 cup ketchup
- 2 eggs

Directions:

1. Switch on the grill, fill the grill hopper with Texas beef blend flavored wood pellets, power the grill on by using the control panel, select 'smoke' on the temperature dial, or set the temperature to 225 degrees F and let it preheat for a minimum of 5 minutes.

2. Meanwhile, take a large bowl, place all the ingredients in it except for ketchup and then stir until well combined.

3. Shape the mixture into meatloaf and then sprinkle with some BBQ rub.

4. When the grill has preheated, open the lid, place meatloaf on the grill grate, shut the grill, and smoke for 2 hours and 15 minutes.

5. Then change the smoking temperature to 375 degrees F, insert a food thermometer into the meatloaf and cook for 45 minutes or more until the internal temperature of meatloaf reaches 155 degrees F.

6. Brush the top of meatloaf with ketchup and then continue cooking for 15 minutes until glazed. When done, transfer food to a dish, let it rest for 10 minutes, then cut it into slices and serve.

Nutrition Info: Calories: 160.5 Cal ;Fat: 2.8 g ;Carbs: 13.2 g ;Protein: 17.2 g ;Fiber: 1 g

St. Louis Bbq Ribs

Servings: 4-6

Cooking Time: 4 Hours 20 Minutes

Ingredients:

- pork as well as a poultry rub - 6 oz
- St. Louis bone in the form of pork ribs - 2 racks
- Heat and Sweet BBQ sauce - 1 bottle
- Apple juice - 8 oz

Directions:

1. Trim the ribs and peel off their membranes from the back.

2. Apply an even coat of the poultry rub on the front and back of the ribs. Let the coat sit for at least 20 minutes. If you wish to refrigerate it, you can do so for up to 4 hours.

3. Once you are ready to cook it, preheat the pellet grill for around 15 minutes. Place the ribs on the grill grate, bone side down. Put the apple juice in an easy spray bottle and then spray it evenly on the ribs.

4. Smoke the meat for 1 hour.

5. Remove the ribs from the pellet grill and wrap them securely in aluminum foil. Ensure that there is an opening in the wrapping at one end. Pour the remaining 6 oz of apple juice into the foil. Wrap it tightly.

6. Place the ribs on the grill again, meat side down. Smoke the meat for another 3 hours.

7. Once the ribs are done and cooked evenly, get rid of the foil. Gently brush a layer of the sauce on both sides of the ribs. Put them back on the grill to cook for another 10 minutes to ensure that the sauce is set correctly.

8. Once the sauce sets, take the ribs off the pellet grill and rest for at least 10 minutes to soak in all the juices.

9. Slice the ribs to serve and enjoy!

Nutrition Info: Carbohydrates: 13 g Protein: 67 g Fat: 70 g Sodium: 410 mg Cholesterol: 180 mg

The Perfect T-bones

Servings: 4

Cooking Time: 30 Minutes

Ingredients:

- 4 (1½- to 2-inch-thick) T-bone steaks
- 2 tablespoons olive oil
- 1 batch Espresso Brisket Rub or Chili-Coffee Rub

Directions:

1. Supply your with wood pellets and follow the start-up procedure. Preheat the grill, with the lid closed, to 500°F.
2. Coat the steaks all over with olive oil and season both sides with the rub. Using your hands, work the rub into the meat.
3. Place the steaks directly on a grill grate and smoke until their internal temperature reaches 135°F for rare, 145°F for medium-rare, and 155°F for well-done. Remove the steaks from the grill and serve hot.

Pork Steak

Servings: 4
Cooking Time: 20 Minutes
Ingredients:
- For the Brine:
- 2-inch piece of orange peel
- 2 sprigs of thyme
- 4 tablespoons salt
- 4 black peppercorns
- 1 sprig of rosemary
- 2 tablespoons brown sugar
- 2 bay leaves
- 10 cups water
- For Pork Steaks:
- 4 pork steaks, fat trimmed
- Game rub as needed

Directions:
1. Prepare the brine and for this, take a large container, place all of its ingredients in it and stir until sugar has dissolved.
2. Place steaks in it, add some weights to keep steak submerge into the brine and let soak for 24 hours in the refrigerator.
3. When ready to cook, switch on the grill, fill the grill hopper with hickory flavored wood pellets, power the grill on by using the control panel, select 'smoke' on the temperature dial, or set the temperature to 225 degrees F and let it preheat for a minimum of 15 minutes.
4. Meanwhile, remove steaks from the brine, rinse well, pat dry with paper towels and then season well with game rub until coated.

5. When the grill has preheated, open the lid, place steaks on the grill grate, shut the grill and smoke for 10 minutes per side until the internal temperature reaches the 140 degrees F.
6. When done, transfer steaks to a cutting board, let them rest for 10 minutes, then cut into slices and serve.
Nutrition Info: Calories: 260 Cal ;Fat: 21 g ;Carbs: 1 g ;Protein: 17 g ;Fiber: 0 g

Wood Pellet Smoked Leg Of lamb

Servings: 6
Cooking Time: 3 Hours
Ingredients:
- 1 leg lamb, boneless
- 4 garlic cloves, minced
- 2 tbsp salt
- 1 tbsp black pepper, freshly ground
- 2 tbsp oregano
- 1 tbsp thyme
- 2 tbsp olive oil

Directions:
1. Trim any excess fat from the lamb and tie the lamb using twine to form a nice roast.
2. In a mixing bowl, mix garlic, spices, and oil. Rub all over the lamb, wrap with a plastic bag then refrigerate for an hour to marinate.
3. Place the lamb on a smoker set at 250 F. smoke the lamb for 4 hours or until the internal temperature reaches 145 F.
4. Remove from the smoker and let rest to cool. Serve and enjoy.
Nutrition Info: Calories 356, Total fat16 g, Saturated fat 5g, Total Carbs 3g, Net Carbs 2g, Protein 49g, Sugar 1g, Fiber 1g, Sodium: 2474mg

Reverse Seared Flank Steak

Servings: 2
Cooking Time: 20 Minutes
Ingredients:
- 3 pound flank steaks
- 1 tbsp salt
- 1/2 tbsp onion powder
- 1/4 tbsp garlic powder

- 1/2 black pepper, coarsely ground

Directions:

1. Preheat the to 225F.
2. Add the steaks and rub them generously with the rub mixture.
3. Place the steak
4. Let cook until its internal temperature is 100F under your desired temperature. 115F for rare, 125F for the medium rear and 135F for medium.
5. Wrap the steak with foil and raise the grill temperature to high. Place back the steak and grill for 3 minutes on each side.
6. Pat with butter and serve when hot.

Nutrition Info: Calories: 112 Cal Fat: 5 g Carbohydrates: 1 g Protein: 16 g Fiber: 0 g

Trager New York Strip

Servings: 6
Cooking Time: 15 Minutes
Ingredients:

- 3 New York strips
- Salt and pepper

Directions:

1. If the steak is in the fridge, remove it 30 minutes prior to cooking.
2. Preheat the to 450F.
3. Meanwhile, season the steak generously with salt and pepper. Place it on the grill and let it cook for 5 minutes per side or until the internal temperature reaches 1280F.
4. Remove the steak from the grill and let it rest for 10 minutes.

Nutrition Info: Calories 198, Total fat 14g, Saturated fat 6g, Total carbs 0g, Net carbs 0g Protein 17g, Sugars 0g, Fiber 0g, Sodium 115mg

Pork Belly

Servings: 8
Cooking Time: 3 Hours And 30 Minutes
Ingredients:

- 3 pounds pork belly, skin removed
- Pork and poultry rub as needed
- 4 tablespoons salt
- 1/2 teaspoon ground black pepper

Directions:

1. Switch on the grill, fill the grill hopper with apple-flavored wood pellets, power the grill on by using the control panel, select 'smoke' on the temperature dial, or set the temperature to 275 degrees F and let it preheat for a minimum of 15 minutes.
2. Meanwhile, prepare the pork belly and for this, sprinkle pork and poultry rub, salt, and black pepper on all sides of pork belly until well coated.
3. When the grill has preheated, open the lid, place the pork belly on the grill grate, shut the grill and smoke for 3 hours and 30 minutes until the internal temperature reaches 200 degrees F.
4. When done, transfer pork belly to a cutting board, let it rest for 15 minutes, then cut it into slices and serve.

Nutrition Info: Calories: 430 Cal ;Fat: 44 g ;Carbs: 1 g ;Protein: 8 g ;Fiber: 0 g

Pineapple Pork Bbq

Servings: 4
Cooking Time: 60 Minutes
Ingredients:

- 1-pound pork sirloin
- 4 cups pineapple juice
- 3 cloves garlic, minced
- 1 cup carne asada marinade
- 2 tablespoons salt
- 1 teaspoon ground black pepper

Directions:

1. Place all ingredients in a bowl. Massage the pork sirloin to coat with all ingredients. Place inside the fridge to marinate for at least 2 hours.
2. When ready to cook, fire the Grill to 300F. Use desired wood pellets when cooking the ribs. Close the lid and preheat for 15 minutes.
3. Place the pork sirloin on the grill grate and cook for 45 to 60 minutes. Make sure to flip the pork halfway through the cooking time.
4. At the same time when you put the pork on the grill grate, place the marinade in a pan and place inside the smoker. Allow the marinade to cook and reduce.

5. Baste the pork sirloin with the reduced marinade before the cooking time ends.

6. Allow to rest before slicing.

Nutrition Info: Calories per serving: 347; Protein: 33.4 g; Carbs: 45.8 g; Fat: 4.2g Sugar: 36g

Braised Elk Shank

Servings: 6
Cooking Time: 4 Hours And 10 Minutes
Ingredients:
- 3 elk shanks
- Salt and pepper to taste
- 3 tablespoons canola oil
- 2 whole onions, halved
- 4 cloves of garlic, minced
- 2 dried bay leaves
- 2 cups red wine
- 1 sprig of rosemary
- 2 carrots, peeled and halved lengthwise
- 1 bunch fresh thyme
- 3 quarts beef stock

Directions:
1. Fire the Grill to 500F. Use desired wood pellets when cooking. Place a cast-iron pan on the grill grate. Close the lid and preheat for 15 minutes.
2. Season the shanks with salt and pepper. Place canola oil in the heated cast iron and place the shanks. Close the grill lid and cook for five minutes on each side.
3. Add the onions and garlic and sauté for 1 minute.
4. Stir in the rest of the ingredients.
5. Close the grill lid and cook for 4 hours until soft.

Nutrition Info: Calories per serving: 331 ;
Protein: 47.2g; Carbs: 11.5g; Fat: 11.2g Sugar: 5.4g

Country Pork Roast

Servings: 8
Cooking Time: 3 Hours
Ingredients:
- 1 (28-ounce) jar or 2 (14.5-ounce) cans sauerkraut
- 3 Granny Smith apples, cored and chopped
- ¾ cup packed light brown sugar
- 3 tablespoons Greek seasoning
- 2 teaspoons dried basil leaves
- Extra-virgin olive oil, for rubbing
- 1 (2- to 2½-pound) pork loin roast

Directions:
1. Supply your smoker with wood pellets and follow the manufacturer's specific start-up procedure. Preheat, with the lid closed, to 250°F.
2. In a large bowl, stir together the sauerkraut, chopped apples, and brown sugar.
3. Spread the sauerkraut-apple mixture in the bottom of a 9-by-13-inch baking dish.
4. In a small bowl, mix together the Greek seasoning and dried basil for the rub.
5. Oil the pork roast and apply the rub, then place it fat-side up in the baking dish, on top of the sauerkraut.
6. Transfer the baking dish to the grill, close the lid, and roast the pork for 3 hours, or until a meat thermometer inserted in the thickest part of the meat reads 160°F.
7. Remove the pork roast from the baking dish and let rest for 5 minutes before slicing.
8. To serve, divide the sauerkraut-apple mixture among plates and top with the sliced pork.

Wood Pellet Togarashi Pork Tenderloin

Servings: 6
Cooking Time: 25 Minutes
Ingredients:
- 1 Pork tenderloin
- 1/2tbsp kosher salt
- 1/4 cup Togarashi seasoning

Directions:
1. Cut any excess silver skin from the pork and sprinkle with salt to taste. Rub generously with the togarashi seasoning
2. Place in a preheated oven at 400°F for 25 minutes or until the internal temperature reaches 145°F.
3. Remove from the grill and let rest for 10 minutes before slicing and serving.
4. Enjoy.

Nutrition Info: Calories 390, Total fat 13g, Saturated fat 6g, Total Carbs 4g, Net Carbs 1g, Protein 33g, Sugar 0g, Fiber 3g, Sodium: 66mg

Texas Smoked Brisket

Servings: 12 To 15

Cooking Time: 16 To 20 Hours

Ingredients:

- 1 (12-pound) full packer brisket
- 2 tablespoons yellow mustard
- 1 batch Espresso Brisket Rub
- Worcestershire Mop and Spritz, for spritzing

Directions:

1. Supply your with wood pellets and follow the start-up procedure. Preheat the grill, with the lid closed, to 225°F.
2. Using a boning knife, carefully remove all but about ½ inch of the large layer of fat covering one side of your brisket.
3. Coat the brisket all over with mustard and season it with the rub. Using your hands, work the rub into the meat. Pour the mop into a spray bottle.
4. Place the brisket directly on the grill grate and smoke until its internal temperature reaches 195°F, spritzing it every hour with the mop.
5. Pull the brisket from the grill and wrap it completely in aluminum foil or butcher paper. Place the wrapped brisket in a cooler, cover the cooler, and let it rest for 1 or 2 hours.
6. Remove the brisket from the cooler and unwrap it.
7. Separate the brisket point from the flat by cutting along the fat layer and slice the flat. The point can be saved for burnt ends (see Sweet Heat Burnt Ends), or sliced and served as well.

Chinese Bbq Pork

Servings: 8

Cooking Time: 2 Hours

Ingredients:

- 2 pork tenderloins, silver skin removed
- For the Marinade:
- ½ teaspoon minced garlic
- 1 1/2 tablespoon brown sugar
- 1 teaspoon Chinese five-spice
- 1/4 cup honey
- 1 tablespoon Asian sesame oil
- 1/4 cup hoisin sauce
- 2 teaspoons red food coloring
- 1 tablespoon oyster sauce, optional
- 3 tablespoons soy sauce
- For the Five-Spice Sauce:
- 1/4 teaspoon Chinese five-spice
- 3 tablespoons brown sugar
- 1 teaspoon yellow mustard
- 1/4 cup ketchup

Directions:

1. Prepare the marinade and for this, take a small bowl, place all of its ingredients in it and whisk until combined.
2. Take a large plastic bag, pour marinade in it, add pork tenderloin, seal the bag, turn it upside down to coat the pork and let it marinate for a minimum of 8 hours in the refrigerator.
3. Switch on the grill, fill the grill hopper with maple-flavored wood pellets, power the grill on by using the control panel, select 'smoke' on the temperature dial, or set the temperature to 225 degrees F and let it preheat for a minimum of 5 minutes.
4. Meanwhile, remove pork from the marinade, transfer marinade into a small saucepan, place it over medium-high heat and cook for 3 minutes, and then set aside until cooled.
5. When the grill has preheated, open the lid, place pork on the grill grate, shut the grill and smoke for 2 hours, basting with the marinade halfway.
6. Meanwhile, prepare the five-spice sauce and for this, take a small saucepan, place it over low heat, add all of its ingredients, stir until well combined and sugar has dissolved and cooked for 5 minutes until hot and thickened, set aside until required.
7. When done, transfer pork to a dish, let rest for 15 minutes, and meanwhile, change the smoking temperature of the grill to 450 degrees F and let it preheat for a minimum of 10 minutes.
8. Then return pork to the grill grate and cook for 3 minutes per side until slightly charred.
9. Transfer pork to a dish, let rest for 5 minutes, and then serve with prepared five-spice sauce.

Nutrition Info: Calories: 280 Cal ;Fat: 8 g ;Carbs: 12 g ;Protein: 40 g ;Fiber: 0 g

Real Treat Chuck Roast

Servings: 8
Cooking Time: 4½ Hours
Ingredients:
- 2 tbsp. onion powder
- 2 tbsp. garlic powder
- 1 tbsp. red chili powder
- 1 tbsp. cayenne pepper
- Salt and freshly ground black pepper, to taste
- 1 (3 lb.) beef chuck roast
- 16 fluid oz. warm beef broth

Directions:
1. Set the temperature of Grill to 250 degrees F and preheat with closed lid for 15 minutes.
2. In a bowl, mix together spices, salt and black pepper.
3. Rub the chuck roast with spice mixture evenly.
4. Place the rump roast onto the grill and cook for about 1½ hours per side.
5. Now, arrange chuck roast in a steaming pan with beef broth.
6. With a piece of foil, cover the pan and cook for about 2-3 hours.
7. Remove the chuck roast from grill and place onto a cutting board for about 20 minutes before slicing.
8. With a sharp knife, cut the chuck roast into desired-sized slices and serve.
Nutrition Info: Calories per serving: 645; Carbohydrates: 4.2g; Protein: 46.4g; Fat: 48g; Sugar: 1.4g; Sodium: 329mg; Fiber: 1g

Wood Pellet Grilled Shredded Pork Tacos

Servings: 8
Cooking Time: 7 Hours
Ingredients:
- 5 lb pork shoulder, bone-in
- Dry Rub
- 3 tbsp brown sugar
- 1 tbsp salt
- 1 tbsp garlic powder
- 1 tbsp paprika
- 1 tbsp onion powder
- 1/4 tbsp cumin
- 1 tbsp cayenne pepper

Directions:
1. Mix all the dry rub ingredients and rub on the pork shoulder.
2. Preheat the grill to 275°F and cook the pork directly for 6 hours or until the internal temperature has reached 145°F.
3. If you want to fall off the bone tender pork, then cook until the internal temperature is 190°F.
4. Let rest for 10 minutes before serving. Enjoy
Nutrition Info: Calories 566, Total fat 41g, Saturated fat 15g, Total Carbs 4g, Net Carbs 4g, Protein 44g, Sugar 3g, Fiber 0g, Sodium: 659mg

Smoked And Pulled Beef

Servings: 6
Cooking Time: 6 Hours
Ingredients:
- 4 lb beef sirloin tip roast
- 1/2 cup bbq rub
- 2 bottles of amber beer
- 1 bottle barbecues sauce

Directions:
1. Turn your wood pellet grill onto smoke setting then trim excess fat from the steak.
2. Coat the steak with bbq rub and let it smoke on the grill for 1 hour.
3. Continue cooking and flipping the steak for the next 3 hours. Transfer the steak to a braising vessel .add the beers.
4. Braise the beef until tender then transfer to a platter reserving 2 cups of cooking liquid.
5. Use a pair of forks to shred the beef and return it to the pan. Add the reserved liquid and barbecue sauce. Stir well and keep warm before serving.
6. Enjoy.
Nutrition Info: Calories 829, Total fat 46g, Saturated fat 18g, Total carbs 4g, Net carbs 4g, Protein 86g, Sugar 0g, Fiber 0g, Sodium: 181mg

Cowboy Steak

Servings: 4
Cooking Time: 1 Hour
Ingredients:
- 2.5 lb. cowboy cut steaks

- Salt to taste
- Beef rub
- 1/4 cup olive oil
- 2 tablespoons fresh mint leaves, chopped
- ½ cup parsley, chopped
- 1 clove garlic, crushed and minced
- 1 tablespoon lemon juice
- 1 tablespoon lemon zest
- Salt and pepper to taste

Directions:

1. Season the steak with the salt and dry rub.
2. Preheat the wood pellet grill to 225 degrees F for 10 minutes while the lid is closed.
3. Grill the steaks for 45 minutes, flipping once or twice.
4. Increase temperature to 450 degrees F.
5. Put the steaks back to the grill. Cook for 5 minutes per side.
6. In a bowl, mix the remaining ingredients.
7. Serve steaks with the parsley mixture.
8. Tips: Let steak rest for 10 minutes before putting it back to the grill for the second round of cooking.

Citrus-brined Pork Roast

Servings: 6
Cooking Time: 45 Minutes
Ingredients:

- ½ cup salt
- ¼ cup brown sugar
- 3 cloves of garlic, minced
- 2 dried bay leaves
- 6 peppercorns
- 1 lemon, juiced
- ½ teaspoon dried fennel seeds
- ½ teaspoon red pepper flakes
- ½ cup apple juice
- ½ cup orange juice
- 5 pounds pork loin
- 2 tablespoons extra virgin olive oil

Directions:

1. In a bowl, combine the salt, brown sugar, garlic, bay leaves, peppercorns, lemon juice, fennel seeds, pepper flakes, apple juice, and orange juice. Mix to form a paste rub.

2. Rub the mixture on to the pork loin and allow to marinate for at least 2 hours in the fridge. Add in the oil.
3. When ready to cook, fire the Grill to 300F. Use apple wood pellets when cooking. Close the lid and preheat for 15 minutes.
4. Place the seasoned pork loin on the grill grate and close the lid. Cook for 45 minutes. Make sure to flip the pork halfway through the cooking time.

Nutrition Info: Calories per serving: 869; Protein: 97.2g; Carbs: 15.2g; Fat: 43.9g Sugar: 13g

Smoked Pork Sausages

Servings: 6
Cooking Time: 1 Hour
Ingredients:

- 3 pounds ground pork
- ½ tablespoon ground mustard
- 1 tablespoon onion powder
- 1 tablespoon garlic powder
- 1 teaspoon pink curing salt
- 1 teaspoon salt
- 1 teaspoon black pepper
- ¼ cup ice water
- Hog casings, soaked and rinsed in cold water

Directions:

1. Mix all ingredients except for the hog casings in a bowl. Using your hands, mix until all ingredients are well-combined.
2. Using a sausage stuffer, stuff the hog casings with the pork mixture.
3. Measure 4 inches of the stuffed hog casing and twist to form into a sausage. Repeat the process until you create sausage links.
4. When ready to cook, fire the Grill to 225F. Use apple wood pellets when cooking the ribs. Close the lid and preheat for 15 minutes.
5. Place the sausage links on the grill grate and cook for 1 hour or until the internal temperature of the sausage reads at 155F.
6. Allow to rest before slicing.

Nutrition Info: Calories per serving: 688; Protein: 58.9g; Carbs: 2.7g; Fat: 47.3g Sugar: 0.2g

Beef Shoulder Clod

Servings: 16-20
Cooking Time: 12-16 Hours
Ingredients:
- ½ cup sea salt
- ½ cup freshly ground black pepper
- 1 tablespoon red pepper flakes
- 1 tablespoon minced garlic
- 1 tablespoon cayenne pepper
- 1 tablespoon smoked paprika
- 1 (13- to 15-pound) beef shoulder clod

Directions:
1. Combine spices
2. Generously apply it to the beef shoulder.
3. Supply your smoker with wood pellets and follow the manufacturer's specific start-up procedure. Preheat, with the lid closed, to 250°F.
4. Put the meat on the grill grate, close the lid, and smoke for 12 to 16 hours, or until a meat thermometer inserted deeply into the beef reads 195°F. You may need to cover the clod with aluminum foil toward the end of smoking to prevent overbrowning.
5. Let the meat rest and serve

Nutrition Info: Calories: 290 Cal Fat: 22 g Carbohydrates: 0 g Protein: 20 g Fiber: 0 g

Strip Steak With Onion Sauce

Servings: 4
Cooking Time: 1 Hour
Ingredients:
- 2 New York strip steaks
- Prime rib rub
- ½ lb. bacon, chopped
- 1 onion, sliced
- 1/4 cup brown sugar
- 1/2 tablespoon balsamic vinegar
- 3 tablespoons brewed coffee
- 1/4 cup apple juice

Directions:
1. Sprinkle both sides of steaks with prime rib rub.
2. Set the wood pellet grill to 350 degrees F.
3. Preheat for 15 minutes while the lid is closed.
4. Place a pan over the grill.
5. Cook the bacon until crispy.
6. Transfer to a plate.
7. Cook the onion in the bacon drippings for 10 minutes.
8. Stir in brown sugar and cook for 20 minutes.
9. Add the rest of the ingredients and cook for 20 minutes.
10. Grill the steaks for 5 minutes per side.
11. Serve with the onion and bacon mixture.
12. Tips: Ensure steak is in room temperature before seasoning.

Grilled Cuban Pork Chops

Servings: 4
Cooking Time: 7-8 Minutes
Ingredients:
- 4 thick-cut pork chops
- 1/3 cup extra virgin olive oil
- 1/2orange, zest only
- 1cup orange juice * freshly squeezed
- 1lime, zest
- 1cup cilantro, finely chopped
- 1/4 cup mint leaves, chopped
- 4 cloves garlic, minced
- 2- inch ginger, minced
- 2teaspoons dried oregano
- 2teaspoons ground cumin

Directions:
1. Take a large mixing bowl and combine lime juice, lime zest, orange zest, olive oil, cilantro, oregano, cumin, ginger, and garlic.
2. Reserve about ¼ cup of this marinade for further use.
3. Pour this marinates in a large mixing bowl and adds pork chops into the marinade for marinating.
4. Marinate the pork chop for 6 hours.
5. Now insert the grill grate into the grill and close the lid
6. Preheat at high temperature for 10 minutes.
7. After preheating the grill add pork chops to the grill grate and cook for about 7 minutes at medium heat.
8. After half time passes, open the unit and flip the chops to cook for another side.
9. Internal temperature should be 150 degrees F at the end of cooking.

10. Once done, serve.

Nutrition Info: Calories: 478 Total Fat: 33.3g Saturated Fat: 8.5g Cholesterol: 80mg Sodium: 267mg Total Carbohydrate: 13.6g Dietary Fiber 2.2g Total Sugars: 7.6g Protein: 35.5g

Garlic Rack Of Lamb

Servings: 4
Cooking Time: 3 Hours
Ingredients:
- 1 rack of lamb, membrane removed
- For the Marinade:
- 2 teaspoons minced garlic
- 1 teaspoon dried basil
- 1/3 cup cream sherry
- 1 teaspoon dried oregano
- 1/3 cup Marsala wine
- 1 teaspoon dried rosemary
- ½ teaspoon ground black pepper
- 1/3 cup balsamic vinegar
- 2 tablespoons olive oil

Directions:
1. Prepare the marinade and for this, take a small bowl, place all of its ingredients in it and stir until well combined.
2. Place lamb rack in a large plastic bag, pour in marinade, seal the bag, turn it upside down to coat lamb with the marinade and let it marinate for a minimum of 45 minutes in the refrigerator.
3. When ready to cook, switch on the grill, fill the grill hopper with flavored wood pellets, power the grill on by using the control panel, select 'smoke' on the temperature dial, or set the temperature to 250 degrees F and let it preheat for a minimum of 5 minutes.
4. Meanwhile,
5. When the grill has preheated, open the lid, place lamb rack on the grill grate, shut the grill, and smoke for 3 hours until the internal temperature reaches 165 degrees F.
6. When done, transfer lamb rack to a cutting board, let it rest for 10 minutes, then cut into slices and serve.

Nutrition Info: Calories: 210 Cal ;Fat: 11 g ;Carbs: 3 g ;Protein: 25 g ;Fiber: 1 g

Versatile Beef Tenderloin

Servings: 6
Cooking Time: 2 Hours 5 Minutes
Ingredients:
- For Brandy Butter:
- ½ C. butter
- 1 oz. brandy
- For Brandy Sauce:
- 2 oz. brandy
- 8 garlic cloves, minced
- ¼ C. mixed fresh herbs (parsley, rosemary and thyme), chopped
- 2 tsp. honey
- 2 tsp. hot English mustard
- For Tenderloin:
- 1 (2-lb.) center-cut beef tenderloin
- Salt and cracked black peppercorns, to taste

Directions:
1. Set the temperature of Grill to 230 degrees F and preheat with closed lid for 15 minutes.
2. For brandy butter: in a pan, melt butter over medium-low heat.
3. Stir in brandy and remove from heat.
4. Set aside, covered to keep warm.
5. For brandy sauce: in a bowl, add all ingredients and mix until well combined.
6. Season the tenderloin with salt and black peppercorns generously.
7. Coat tenderloin with brandy sauce evenly.
8. With a baster-injector, inject tenderloin with brandy butter.
9. Place the tenderloin onto the grill and cook for about 1½-2 hours, injecting with brandy butter occasionally.
10. Remove the tenderloin from grill and place onto a cutting board for about 10-15 minutes before serving.
11. With a sharp knife, cut the tenderloin into desired-sized slices and serve.

Nutrition Info: Calories per serving: 496; Carbohydrates: 4.4g; Protein: 44.4g; Fat: 29.3g; Sugar: 2g; Sodium: 240mg; Fiber: 0.7g

Pineapple-pepper Pork Kebabs

Servings: 12 To 15
Cooking Time: 1 To 4 Hours
Ingredients:
- 1 (20-ounce) bottle hoisin sauce
- ½ cup Sriracha
- ¼ cup honey
- ¼ cup apple cider vinegar
- 2 tablespoons canola oil
- 2 teaspoons minced garlic
- 2 teaspoons onion powder
- 1 teaspoon ground ginger
- 1 teaspoon salt
- 1 teaspoon freshly ground black pepper
- 2 pounds thick-cut pork chops or pork loin, cut into 2-inch cubes
- 10 ounces fresh pineapple, cut into chunks
- 1 red onion, cut into wedges
- 1 bag mini sweet peppers, tops removed and seeded
- 12 metal or wooden skewers (soaked in water for 30 minutes if wooden)

Directions:
1. In a small bowl, stir together the hoisin, Sriracha, honey, vinegar, oil, minced garlic, onion powder, ginger, salt, and black pepper to create the marinade. Reserve ¼ cup for basting.
2. Toss the pork cubes, pineapple chunks, onion wedges, and mini peppers in the remaining marinade. Cover and refrigerate for at least 1 hour or up to 4 hours.
3. Supply your smoker with wood pellets and follow the manufacturer's specific start-up procedure. Preheat, with the lid closed, to 450°F.
4. Remove the pork, pineapple, and veggies from the marinade; do not rinse. Discard the marinade.
5. Use the double-skewer technique to assemble the kebabs (see Tip below). Thread each of 6 skewers with a piece of pork, a piece of pineapple, a piece of onion, and a sweet mini pepper, making sure that the skewer goes through the left side of the ingredients. Repeat the threading on each skewer two more times. Double-skewer the kebabs by sticking another 6 skewers through the right side of the ingredients.
6. Place the kebabs directly on the grill, close the lid, and smoke for 10 to 12 minutes, turning once.

They are done when a meat thermometer inserted in the pork reads 160°F.

Beef Jerky

Servings: 10
Cooking Time: 5 Hours
Ingredients:
- 3 pounds sirloin steaks
- 2 cups soy sauce
- 1 cup pineapple juice
- 1/2 cup brown sugar
- 2 tbsp sriracha
- 2 tbsp hoisin
- 2 tbsp red pepper flake
- 2 tbsp rice wine vinegar
- 2 tbsp onion powder

Directions:
1. Mix the marinade in a zip lock bag and add the beef. Mix until well coated and remove as much air as possible.
2. Place the bag in a fridge and let marinate overnight or for 6 hours. Remove the bag from the fridge an hour prior to cooking
3. Startup the and set it on the smoking settings or at 190F.
4. Lay the meat on the grill leaving a half-inch space between the pieces. Let cool for 5 hours and turn after 2 hours.
5. Remove from the grill and let cool. Serve or refrigerate
Nutrition Info: Calories: 309 Cal Fat: 7 g Carbohydrates: 20 g   Protein: 34 g Fiber: 1 g

Smoked, Candied, And Spicy Bacon

Servings: 10
Cooking Time: 40 Minutes
Ingredients:
- Center-cut bacon - 1 lb.
- Brown sugar - ½ cup
- Maple syrup - ½ cup
- Hot sauce - 1 tbsp
- Pepper - ½ tbsp
Directions:

1. Mix the maple syrup, brown sugar, hot sauce, and pepper in a bowl.
2. Preheat your wood pellet grill to 300 degrees.
3. Line a baking sheet and place the bacon slices on it.
4. Generously spread the brown sugar mix on both sides of the bacon slices.
5. Place the pan on the wood pellet grill for 20 minutes. Flip the bacon pieces.
6. Leave them for another 15 minutes until the bacon looks cooked, and the sugar is melted.
7. Remove from the grill and let it stay for 10-15 minutes.
8. Voila! Your bacon candy is ready!
Nutrition Info: Carbohydrates: 37 g Protein: 9 g Sodium: 565 mg Cholesterol: 49 mg

Elegant Lamb Chops

Servings: 4
Cooking Time: 30 Minutes
Ingredients:
- 4 lamb shoulder chops
- 4 C. buttermilk
- 1 C. cold water
- ¼ C. kosher salt
- 2 tbsp. olive oil
- 1 tbsp. Texas-style rub

Directions:
1. In a large bowl, add buttermilk, water and salt and stir until salt is dissolved.
2. Add chops and coat with mixture evenly.
3. Refrigerate for at least 4 hours.
4. Remove the chops from bowl and rinse under cold running water.
5. Coat the chops with olive oil and then sprinkle with rub evenly.
6. Set the temperature of Grill to 240 degrees F and preheat with closed lid for 15 minutes, using charcoal.
7. Arrange the chops onto grill and cook for about 25-30 minutes or until desired doneness.
8. Meanwhile, preheat the broiler of oven. Grease a broiler pan.
9. Remove the chops from grill and place onto the prepared broiler pan.

10. Transfer the broiler pan into the oven and broil for about 3-5 minutes or until browned.
11. Remove the chops from oven and serve hot.
Nutrition Info: Calories per serving: 414; Carbohydrates: 11.7g; Protein: 5.6g; Fat: 22.7g; Sugar: 11.7g; Sodium: 7000mg; Fiber: 0g

Lamb Shank

Servings: 6
Cooking Time: 4 Hours
Ingredients:
- 8-ounce red wine
- 2-ounce whiskey
- 2 tablespoons minced fresh rosemary
- 1 tablespoon minced garlic
- Black pepper
- 6 (1¼-pound) lamb shanks

Directions:
1. In a bowl, add all ingredients except lamb shank and mix till well combined.
2. In a large resealable bag, add marinade and lamb shank.
3. Seal the bag and shake to coat completely.
4. Refrigerate for about 24 hours.
5. Preheat the pallet grill to 225 degrees F.
6. Arrange the leg of lamb in pallet grill and cook for about 4 hours.
Nutrition Info: Calories: 1507 Cal Fat: 62 g Carbohydrates: 68.7 g Protein:163.3 g Fiber: 6 g

Mesquite Smoked Brisket

Servings: 8 To 12
Cooking Time: 12 To 16 Hours
Ingredients:
- 1 (12-pound) full packer brisket
- 2 tablespoons yellow mustard (you can also use soy sauce)
- Salt
- Freshly ground black pepper

Directions:
1. Supply your with wood pellets and follow the start-up procedure. Preheat the grill, with the lid closed, to 225°F.

2. Using a boning knife, carefully remove all but about ½ inch of the large layer of fat covering one side of your brisket.

3. Coat the brisket all over with mustard and season it with salt and pepper.

4. Place the brisket directly on the grill grate and smoke until its internal temperature reaches 160°F and the brisket has formed a dark bark.

5. Pull the brisket from the grill and wrap it completely in aluminum foil or butcher paper.

6. Increase the grill's temperature to 350°F and return the wrapped brisket to it. Continue to cook until its internal temperature reaches 190°F.

7. Transfer the wrapped brisket to a cooler, cover the cooler, and let the brisket rest for 1 or 2 hours.

8. Remove the brisket from the cooler and unwrap it.

9. Separate the brisket point from the flat by cutting along the fat layer, and slice the flat. The point can be saved for burnt ends (see Sweet Heat Burnt Ends), or sliced and served as well.

Bbq Baby Back Ribs

Servings: 8
Cooking Time: 6 Hours
Ingredients:
- 2 racks of baby back pork ribs, membrane removed
- Pork and poultry rub as needed
- 1/2 cup brown sugar
- 1/3 cup honey, warmed
- 1/3 cup yellow mustard
- 1 tablespoon Worcestershire sauce
- 1 cup BBQ sauce
- 1/2 cup apple juice, divided

Directions:
1. Switch on the grill, fill the grill hopper with hickory flavored wood pellets, power the grill on by using the control panel, select 'smoke' on the temperature dial, or set the temperature to 180 degrees F and let it preheat for a minimum of 15 minutes.

2. Meanwhile, take a small bowl, place mustard, and Worcestershire sauce in it, pour in ¼ cup apple juice and whisk until combined and smooth paste comes together.

3. Brush this paste on all sides of ribs and then season with pork and poultry rub until coated.

4. When the grill has preheated, open the lid, place ribs on the grill grate meat-side up, shut the grill and smoke for 3 hours.

5. After 3 hours, transfer ribs to a rimmed baking dish, let rest for 15 minutes, and meanwhile, change the smoking temperature of the grill to 225 degrees F and let it preheat for a minimum of 10 minutes.

6. Then return pork into the rimmed baking sheet to the grill grate and cook for 3 minutes per side until slightly charred.

7. When done, remove the baking sheet from the grill and work on one rib at a time, sprinkle half of the sugar over the rib, drizzle with half of the honey and half of the remaining apple juice, cover with aluminum foil to seal completely.

8. Repeat with the remaining ribs, return foiled ribs on the grill grate, shut with lid, and then smoke for 2 hours.

9. After 2 hours, uncover the grill, brush them with BBQ sauce generously, arrange them on the grill grate and grill for 1 hour until glazed.

10. When done, transfer ribs to a cutting board, let it rest for 15 minutes, slice into pieces and then serve.

Nutrition Info: Calories: 334 Cal ;Fat: 22.5 g ;Carbs: 6.5 g ;Protein: 24 g ;Fiber: 0.1 g

Sweet & Spicy Pork Roast

Servings: 4
Cooking Time: 1 Hour And 30 Minutes
Ingredients:
- 3 lb. pork loin
- 1/2 teaspoon Chinese 5 spice
- 1 can coconut milk
- 1 habanero pepper
- 1 teaspoon curry powder
- 1 tablespoon paprika
- 1 teaspoon ginger, grated
- 1 tablespoon garlic, minced
- 1 tablespoon lime juice

Directions:
1. Place pork in a bowl.

2. In another bowl, combine the remaining ingredients.

3. Pour the mixture over the pork and marinate overnight covered in the refrigerator.

4. Set the wood pellet grill to 300 degrees F.

5. Preheat for 15 minutes while the lid is closed.

6. Add the pork to the grill.

7. Cook for 1 hour.

8. Flip and cook for another 30 minutes.

9. Tips: You can also marinate for at least 4 hours.

Stunning Prime Rib Roast

Servings: 10
Cooking Time: 3 Hours 50 Minutes
Ingredients:

- 1 (5-lb.) prime rib roast
- Salt, to taste
- 5 tbsp. olive oil
- 4 tsp. dried rosemary, crushed
- 2 tsp. garlic powder
- 1 tsp. onion powder
- 1 tsp. paprika
- ½ tsp. cayenne pepper
- Freshly ground black pepper, to taste

Directions:

1. Season the roast with salt generously.

2. With a plastic wrap, cover the roast and refrigerate for about 24 hours.

3. In a bowl, mix together remaining ingredients and set aside for about 1 hour.

4. Rub the roast with oil mixture from both sides evenly.

5. Arrange the roast in a large baking sheet and refrigerate for about 6-12 hours.

6. Set the temperature of Grill to 225-230 degrees F and preheat with closed lid for 15 minutes. , using pecan wood chips.

7. Place the roast onto the grill and cook for about 3-3½ hours.

8. Meanwhile, preheat the oven to 500 degrees F.

9. Remove the roast from grill and place onto a large baking sheet.

10. Place the baking sheet in oven and roast for about 15-20 minutes.

11. Remove the roast from oven and place onto a cutting board for about 10-15 minutes before serving.

12. With a sharp knife, cut the roast into desired-sized slices and serve.

Nutrition Info: Calories per serving: 605; Carbohydrates: 3.8g; Protein: 38g; Fat: 47.6g; Sugar: 0.3g; Sodium: 1285mg; Fiber: 0.3g Stunning Prime Rib Roast

Citrus Pork Chops

Servings: 4
Cooking Time: 30 Minutes
Ingredients:

- 2 oranges, sliced into wedges
- 2 lemons, sliced into wedges
- 6 sprigs rosemary, chopped
- 2 sticks butter, softened
- 1 clove garlic, minced
- 4 tablespoons fresh thyme leaves, chopped
- 1 teaspoon black pepper
- 5 pork chops

Directions:

1. Set the wood pellet grill to smoke.

2. Wait for it to establish fire for 5 minutes.

3. Set temperature to high.

4. Squeeze lemons and oranges into a bowl.

5. Stir in the rest of the ingredients except the pork chops.

6. Marinate the pork chops in the mixture for 3 hours.

7. Grill for 10 minutes per side.

8. Tips: Use bone-in pork chops for this recipe.

Southern Sugar-glazed Ham

Servings: 12 To 15
Cooking Time: 5 Hours
Ingredients:

- 1 (12- to 15-pound) whole bone-in ham, fully cooked
- ¼ cup yellow mustard
- 1 cup pineapple juice
- ½ cup packed light brown sugar
- 1 teaspoon ground cinnamon
- ½ teaspoon ground cloves

Directions:

1. Supply your smoker with wood pellets and follow the manufacturer's specific start-up procedure. Preheat, with the lid closed, to 275°F.

2. Trim off the excess fat and skin from the ham, leaving a ¼-inch layer of fat. Put the ham in an aluminum foil–lined roasting pan.

3. On your kitchen stove top, in a medium saucepan over low heat, combine the mustard, pineapple juice, brown sugar, cinnamon, and cloves and simmer for 15 minutes, or until thick and reduced by about half.

4. Baste the ham with half of the pineapple–brown sugar syrup, reserving the rest for basting later in the cook.

5. Place the roasting pan on the grill, close the lid, and smoke for 4 hours.

6. Baste the ham with the remaining pineapple–brown sugar syrup and continue smoking with the lid closed for another hour, or until a meat thermometer inserted in the thickest part of the ham reads 140°F.

7. Remove the ham from the grill, tent with foil, and let rest for 20 minutes before carving.

Slow Roasted Shawarma

Servings: 6-8
Cooking Time: 4 Hours 55 Minutes
Ingredients:

- Top sirloin - 5.5 lbs
- Lamb fat - 4.5 lbs
- Boneless, skinless chicken thighs- 5.5 lbs
- Pita bread
- rub - 4 tbsp
- Double skewer - 1
- Large yellow onions - 2
- Variety of topping options such as tomatoes, cucumbers, pickles, tahini, Israeli salad, fries, etc.
- Cast iron griddle

Directions:

1. Assemble the stack of shawarma the night before you wish to cook it.

2. Slice all the meat and fat into ½-inch slices. Place them into 3 bowls. If you partially freeze them, it will be much easier to slice them.

3. Season the bowl with the rub, massaging it thoroughly into the meat.

4. Place half a yellow onion on the bottom of the skewers to ensure a firm base. Add 2 layers at a time from each bowl. Try to make the entire stack symmetrical. Place the other 2 onions on top. Wrap them in plastic wrap and refrigerate overnight.

5. When the meat is ready to cook, preheat the pellet grill for about 15 minutes with the lid closed at a temperature of 275 degrees Fahrenheit.

6. Lay the shawarma directly on the grill grate and cook it for at least 3-4 hours. Rotate the skewers at least once.

7. Remove them from the grill and increase its temperature to 445 degrees Fahrenheit. When the grill is preheating, place a cast iron griddle directly on the grill grate and brush it with some olive oil.

8. Once the griddle is hot enough, place the shawarma directly on the cast iron. Sear it on each side for 5-10 minutes. Remove it from the grill and slice off the edges. Repeat the process with the remaining shawarma.

9. Serve in pita bread and favorite toppings, such as tomatoes, cucumbers, Israeli salad, fries, pickles, or tahini. Enjoy!

Nutrition Info: Carbohydrates: 4.6 g Protein: 30.3 g Fat: 26.3 g Sodium: 318.7 mg Cholesterol: 125.5 mg

Cowboy Cut Steak

Servings: 4
Cooking Time: 1 Hour And 15 Minutes
Ingredients:

- 2 cowboy cut steak, each about 2 ½ pounds
- Salt as needed
- Beef rub as needed
- For the Gremolata:
- 2 tablespoons chopped mint
- 1 bunch of parsley, leaves separated
- 1 lemon, juiced
- 1 tablespoon lemon zest
- ½ teaspoon minced garlic
- ¼ teaspoon salt
- 1/8 teaspoon ground black pepper
- 1/4 cup olive oil

Directions:

1. Switch on the grill, fill the grill hopper with mesquite flavored wood pellets, power the grill on by using the control panel, select 'smoke' on the temperature dial, or set the temperature to 225 degrees F and let it preheat for a minimum of 5 minutes.

2. Meanwhile, prepare the steaks, and for this, season them with salt and BBQ rub until well coated.

3. When the grill has preheated, open the lid, place steaks on the grill grate, shut the grill and smoke for 45 minutes to 1 hour until thoroughly cooked, and internal temperature reaches 115 degrees F.

4. Meanwhile, prepare gremolata and for this, take a medium bowl, place all of its ingredients in it and then stir well until combined, set aside until combined.

5. When done, transfer steaks to a dish, let rest for 15 minutes, and meanwhile, change the smoking temperature of the grill to 450 degrees F and let it preheat for a minimum of 10 minutes.

6. Then return steaks to the grill grate and cook for 7 minutes per side until the internal temperature reaches 130 degrees F.

Nutrition Info: Calories: 361 Cal ;Fat: 31 g ;Carbs: 1 g ;Protein: 19 g ;Fiber: 0.2 g

Braised Lamb

Servings: 4
Cooking Time: 3 Hours And 20 Minutes
Ingredients:

- 4 lamb shanks
- Prime rib rub
- 1 cup red wine
- 1 cup beef broth
- 2 sprigs thyme
- 2 sprigs rosemary

Directions:

1. Sprinkle all sides of lamb shanks with prime rib rub.

2. Set temperature of the wood pellet grill to high.

3. Preheat it for 15 minutes while the lid is closed.

4. Add the lamb to the grill and cook for 20 minutes.

5. Transfer the lamb to a Dutch oven.

6. Stir in the rest of the ingredients.

7. Transfer back to the grill.

8. Reduce temperature to 325 degrees F.

9. Braise the lamb for 3 hours.

10. Tips: Let cool before serving.

Drunken Beef Jerky

Servings: 6
Cooking Time: 5 Hours
Ingredients:

- 1 (12-oz.) bottle dark beer
- 1 C. soy sauce
- ¼ C. Worcestershire sauce
- 2 tbsp. hot sauce
- 3 tbsp. brown sugar
- 2 tbsp. coarse ground black pepper, divided
- 1 tbsp. curing salt
- ½ tsp. garlic salt
- 2 lb. flank steak, trimmed and cut into ¼-inch thick slices

Directions:

1. In a bowl, add the beer, soy sauce, Worcestershire sauce, brown sugar, 2 tbsp. of black pepper, curing salt and garlic salt and mix well.

2. In a large resealable plastic bag, place the steak slices and marinade mixture.

3. Seal the bag, squeezing out the air and then shake to coat well.

4. Refrigerate to marinate overnight.

5. Set the temperature of Grill to 180 degrees F and preheat with closed lid for 15 minutes.

6. Remove the steak slices from the bag and discard the marinade.

7. With paper towels, pat dry the steak slices.

8. Sprinkle the steak slices with remaining black pepper generously.

9. Arrange the steak slices onto the grill in a single layer and cook for about 4-5 hours.

Nutrition Info: Calories per serving: 374; Carbohydrates: 13.3g; Protein: 45.3g; Fat: 12.7g; Sugar: 7.2g; Sodium: 2700mg; Fiber: 0.9g

Spicy & Tangy Lamb Shoulder

Servings: 6
Cooking Time: 5¾ Hours

Ingredients:
- 1 (5-lb.) bone-in lamb shoulder, trimmed
- 3-4 tbsp. Moroccan seasoning
- 2 tbsp. olive oil
- 1 C. water
- ¼ C. apple cider vinegar

Directions:
1. Set the temperature of Grill to 275 degrees F and preheat with closed lid for 15 minutes, using charcoal.
2. Coat the lamb shoulder with oil evenly and then rub with Moroccan seasoning generously.
3. Place the lamb shoulder onto the grill and cook for about 45 minutes.
4. In a food-safe spray bottle, mix together vinegar and water.
5. Spray the lamb shoulder with vinegar mixture evenly.
6. Cook for about 4-5 hours, spraying with vinegar mixture after every 20 minutes.
7. Remove the lamb shoulder from grill and place onto a cutting board for about 20 minutes before slicing.
8. With a sharp knife, cut the lamb shoulder in desired sized slices and serve.

Nutrition Info: Calories per serving: 563; Carbohydrates: 3.1g; Protein: 77.4g; Fat: 25.2g; Sugar: 1.4g; Sodium: 1192mg; Fiber: 0g

Kalbi Beef Ribs

Servings: 6
Cooking Time: 23 Minutes
Ingredients:
- Thinly sliced beef ribs - 2 ½ lbs
- Soy sauce - ½ cup
- Brown sugar - ½ cup
- Rice wine or mirin - ⅛ cup
- Minced garlic - 2 tbsp
- Sesame oil - 1 tbsp
- Grated onion - ⅛ cup

Directions:
1. In a medium-sized bowl, mix the mirin, soy sauce, sesame oil, brown sugar, garlic, and grated onion.

2. Add the ribs to the bowl to marinate and cover it properly with cling wrap. Put it in the refrigerator for up to 6 hours.
3. Once you remove the marinated ribs from the refrigerator, immediately put them on the grill. Close the grill quickly, so no heat is lost. Also, make sure the grill is preheated well before you place the ribs on it.
4. Cook on one side for 4 minutes and then flip it. Cook the other side for 4 minutes.
5. Pull it out once it looks fully cooked. Serve it with rice or any other side dish

Nutrition Info: Carbohydrates: 22 g Protein: 28 g Fat: 6 g Sodium: 1213 mg Cholesterol: 81 mg

French Onion Burgers

Servings: 4
Cooking Time: 20-25 Minutes
Ingredients:
- 1-pound lean ground beef
- 1 tablespoon minced garlic
- 1 teaspoon Better Than Bouillon Beef Base
- 1 teaspoon dried chives
- 1 teaspoon freshly ground black pepper
- 8 slices Gruyère cheese, divided
- ½ cup soy sauce
- 1 tablespoon extra-virgin olive oil
- 1 teaspoon liquid smoke
- 3 medium onions, cut into thick slices (do not separate the rings)
- 1 loaf French bread, cut into 8 slices
- 4 slices provolone cheese

Directions:
1. In a large bowl, mix together the ground beef, minced garlic, beef base, chives, and pepper until well blended.
2. Divide the meat mixture and shape into 8 thin burger patties.
3. Top each of 4 patties with one slice of Gruyère, then top with the remaining 4 patties to create 4 stuffed burgers.
4. Supply your smoker with wood pellets and follow the manufacturer's specific start-up procedure. Preheat, with the lid closed, to 425°F.

5. Arrange the burgers directly on one side of the grill, close the lid, and smoke for 10 minutes. Flip and smoke with the lid closed for 10 to 15 minutes more, or until a meat thermometer inserted in the burgers reads 160°F. Add another Gruyère slice to the burgers during the last 5 minutes of smoking to melt.

6. Meanwhile, in a small bowl, combine the soy sauce, olive oil, and liquid smoke.

7. Arrange the onion slices on the grill and baste on both sides with the soy sauce mixture. Smoke with the lid closed for 20 minutes, flipping halfway through.

8. Lightly toast the French bread slices on the grill. Layer each of 4 slices with a burger patty, a slice of provolone cheese, and some of the smoked onions. Top each with another slice of toasted French bread. Serve immediately.

Nutrition Info: Calories: 704 Cal Fat: 43 g Carbohydrates: 28 g   Protein: 49 g Fiber: 2 g

Sweet Smoked Country Ribs

Servings: 12 To 15
Cooking Time: 4 Hours
Ingredients:
- 2 pounds country-style ribs
- 1 batch Sweet Brown Sugar Rub
- 2 tablespoons light brown sugar
- 1 cup Pepsi or other cola
- ¼ cup The Ultimate BBQ Sauce

Directions:
1. Supply your smoker with wood pellets and follow the manufacturer's specific start-up procedure. Preheat the grill, with the lid closed, to 180°F.
2. Sprinkle the ribs with the rub and use your hands to work the rub into the meat.
3. Place the ribs directly on the grill grate and smoke for 3 hours.
4. Remove the ribs from the grill and place them on enough aluminum foil to wrap them completely. Dust the brown sugar over the ribs.
5. Increase the grill's temperature to 300°F.
6. Fold in three sides of the foil around the ribs and add the cola. Fold in the last side, completely enclosing the ribs and liquid. Return the ribs to the grill and cook for 45 minutes.

7. Remove the ribs from the foil and place them on the grill grate. Baste all sides of the ribs with barbecue sauce. Cook for 15 minutes more to caramelize the sauce.

8. Remove the ribs from the grill and serve immediately.

Cocoa Crusted Pork Tenderloin

Servings: 5
Cooking Time: 25 Minutes
Ingredients:
- 1 pork tenderloin
- 1/2 tbsp fennel, ground
- 2 tbsp cocoa powder, unsweetened
- 1 tbsp smoked paprika
- 1/2 tbsp kosher salt
- 1/2 tbsp black pepper
- 1 tbsp extra virgin olive oil
- 3 green onion

Directions:
1. Remove the silver skin and the connective tissues from the pork loin.
2. Combine the rest of the ingredients in a mixing bowl, then rub the mixture on the pork. Refrigerate for 30 minutes.
3. Preheat the wood pellet grill for 15 minutes with the lid closed.
4. Sear all sides of the loin at the front of the grill then reduce the temperature to 350°F and move the pork to the centre grill.
5. Cook for 15 more minutes or until the internal temperature is 145°F.
6. Remove from grill and let rest for 10 minutes before slicing. Enjoy

Nutrition Info: Calories 264, Total fat 13.1g, Saturated fat 6g, Total Carbs 4.6g, Net Carbs 1.2g, Protein 33g, Sugar 0g, Fiber 3.4g, Sodium: 66mg

Smoked Pork Tenderloin

Servings: 4-6
Cooking Time: 1 Hour And 30 Minutes
Ingredients:
- 2 (1½2 pounds) pork fillet

- ¼ Extra virgin olive oil with cup roasted garlic flavor
- ¼Cup Jan's Original Dry Rub or Pork Dry Rub

Directions:

1. Configure a wood pellet smoker grill for indirect cooking and preheat to 230 ° F using hickory or apple pellets.
2. Remove the wrap from the meat and insert a wood pellet smoker grill probe or remote meat probe into the thickest part of each tenderloin. If your grill does not have a meat probe or you do not have a remote meat probe, use an instant reading digital thermometer to read the internal temperature while cooking.
3. Place the tenderloin directly on the grill and smoke at 230 ° F for 45 minutes.
4. Raise the temperature of the pit to 350 ° F and finish cooking the tenderloin for about 45 minutes until the internal temperature of the thickest part reaches 145 ° F.
5. Rest the pork tenderloin under a loose foil tent for 10 minutes before serving.

Nutrition Info: Calories: 115 Cal Fat: 3 g Carbohydrates: 0 g   Protein: 22 g Fiber: 0 g

Wood Pellet Grilled Lamb With Brown Sugar Glaze

Servings: 4
Cooking Time: 10 Minutes
Ingredients:

- 1/4 cup brown sugar
- 2 tbsp ginger, ground
- 2 tbsp tarragon, dried
- 1 tbs cinnamon, ground
- 1 tbsp black pepper, ground
- 1 tbsp garlic powder
- 1/2 tbsp salt
- 4 lamb chops

Directions:

1. In a mixing bowl, mix sugar, ginger, dried tarragon, cinnamon, black pepper, garlic, and salt.
2. Rub the lamb chops with the seasoning and place it on a plate.refrigerate for an hour to marinate.
3. Preheat the grill to high heat then brush the grill grate with oil.

4. Arrange the lamb chops on the grill grate in a single layer and cook for 5 minutes on each side.
5. Serve and enjoy.

Nutrition Info: Calories 241, Total fat 13.1g, Saturated fat 6g, Total Carbs 15.8g, Net Carbs 15.1g, Protein 14.6g, Sugar 14g, Fiber 0.7g, Sodium: 339mg,

Smoked Sausages

Servings: 4
Cooking Time: 3 Hours
Ingredients:

- 3 pounds ground pork
- 1 tablespoon onion powder
- 1 tablespoon garlic powder
- 1 teaspoon curing salt
- 4 teaspoon black pepper
- 1/2 tablespoon salt
- 1/2 tablespoon ground mustard
- Hog casings, soaked
- 1/2 cup ice water

Directions:

1. Switch on the grill, fill the grill hopper with flavored wood pellets, power the grill on by using the control panel, select 'smoke' on the temperature dial, or set the temperature to 225 degrees F and let it preheat for a minimum of 15 minutes.
2. Meanwhile, take a medium bowl, place all the ingredients in it except for water and hog casings, and stir until well mixed.
3. Pour in water, stir until incorporated, place the mixture in a sausage stuffer, then stuff the hog casings and tie the link to the desired length.
4. When the grill has preheated, open the lid, place the sausage links on the grill grate, shut the grill, and smoke for 2 to 3 hours until the internal temperature reaches 155 degrees F.
5. When done, transfer sausages to a dish, let them rest for 5 minutes, then slice and serve.

Nutrition Info: Calories: 230 Cal ;Fat: 22 g ;Carbs: 2 g ;Protein: 14 g ;Fiber: 0 g

Bbq Brisket

Servings: 8
Cooking Time: 10 Hours

Ingredients:
- 1 beef brisket, about 12 pounds
- Beef rub as needed

Directions:
1. Season beef brisket with beef rub until well coated, place it in a large plastic bag, seal it and let it marinate for a minimum of 12 hours in the refrigerator.
2. When ready to cook, switch on the grill, fill the grill hopper with hickory flavored wood pellets, power the grill on by using the control panel, select 'smoke' on the temperature dial, or set the temperature to 225 degrees F and let it preheat for a minimum of 15 minutes.
3. When the grill has preheated, open the lid, place marinated brisket on the grill grate fat-side down, shut the grill, and smoke for 6 hours until the internal temperature reaches 160 degrees F.
4. Then wrap the brisket in foil, return it back to the grill grate and cook for 4 hours until the internal temperature reaches 204 degrees F.
5. When done, transfer brisket to a cutting board, let it rest for 30 minutes, then cut it into slices and serve.

Nutrition Info: Calories: 328 Cal ;Fat: 21 g ;Carbs: 0 g ;Protein: 32 g ;Fiber: - g

Asian Steak Skewers

Servings: 6
Cooking Time: 1 Hour And 20 Minutes
Ingredients:
- 1 1/2 lbs top sirloin steak
- 6 garlic cloves, minced
- 1 red onion
- 1/3 cup sugar
- 3/4 cup soy sauce
- 1 tbsp ground ginger
- 1/4 cup sesame oil
- 3 tbsp sesame seeds
- 1/4 cup vegetable oil
- Bamboo skewers

Directions:
1. Cut sirloin steak into cubes, about 1 inch.
2. Cut red onion into chunks similar in size to the sirloin steak cubes.

3. In a bowl, combine and whisk soy sauce, sesame oil, vegetable oil, minced garlic, sugar, ginger, and sesame seeds.
4. Add steak to sauce bowl and toss to coat until steak is covered in the sauce.
5. Marinate for at least 1 hour in a refrigerator (if you are in a rush it's ok to skip this part, but you'll sacrifice a little bit of flavor).
6. Preheat pellet grill to 350°F.
7. Thread marinated beef and red onion pieces onto bamboo skewers.
8. Grill the skewers, turning after about 4 minutes. Cook for 8 minutes total or until meat reaches your desired doneness.

Bacon

Servings: 6
Cooking Time: 25 Minutes
Ingredients:
- 1lb bacon

Directions:
1. Preheat your to 375F.
2. Line a baking sheet with parchment paper then arrange the thick-cut bacon on it in a single layer.
3. Bake the bacon in the for 20 minutes. Flip the bacon pieces and cook for 20 more minutes or until the bacon is no longer floppy.
4. Serve and enjoy.

Nutrition Info: Calories 315, Total fat 10g, Saturated fat 0g, Total carbs 0g, Net carbs 0g Protein 9g, Sugars 0g, Fiber 0g, Sodium 500mg

Smoked Lamb Meatballs

Servings: 5
Cooking Time: 1 Hour
Ingredients:
- 1 lb lamb shoulder, ground
- 3 garlic cloves, finely diced
- 3 tbsp shallot, diced
- 1 tbsp salt
- 1 egg
- 1/2 tbsp pepper
- 1/2 tbsp cumin
- 1/2 tbsp smoked paprika

- 1/4 tbsp red pepper flakes
- 1/4 tbsp cinnamon, ground
- 1/4 cup panko breadcrumbs

Directions:

1. Set the wood pellet smoker to 250 F using a fruitwood.
2. In a mixing bowl, combine all meatball ingredients until well mixed.
3. Form small-sized balls and place them on a baking sheet. Place the baking sheet in the smoker and smoke until the internal temperature reaches 160 F.
4. Remove from the smoker and serve. Enjoy.

Nutrition Info: Calories 73, Total fat 5.2g, Saturated fat 1.6g, Total Carbs 1.5g, Net Carbs 1.4g, Protein 4.9g, Sugar 0g, Fiber 0.1g, Sodium: 149mg, Potassium 72mg

2. On your kitchen stove top, in a large saucepan over high heat, bring the chicken stock and water to a boil.
3. Add the grits and reduce the heat to low, then stir in the butter, garlic, onion, jalapeño, cayenne, red pepper flakes, hot sauce, cheese, and sour cream. Season with salt and pepper, then cook for about 5 minutes.
4. Temper the beaten eggs (see Tip below) and incorporate into the grits. Remove the saucepan from the heat and stir in the half-and-half and pulled pork.
5. Pour the grits into a greased grill-safe 9-by-13-inch casserole dish or aluminum pan.
6. Transfer to the grill, close the lid, and bake for 30 to 40 minutes, covering with aluminum foil toward the end of cooking if the grits start to get too brown on top.

Bbq Breakfast Grits

Servings: 12 To 15
Cooking Time: 30 To 40 Minutes

Ingredients:

- 2 cups chicken stock
- 1 cup water
- 1 cup quick-cooking grits
- 3 tablespoons unsalted butter
- 2 tablespoons minced garlic
- 1 medium onion, chopped
- 1 jalapeño pepper, stemmed, seeded, and chopped
- 1 teaspoon cayenne pepper
- 2 teaspoons red pepper flakes
- 1 tablespoon hot sauce
- 1 cup shredded Monterey Jack cheese
- 1 cup sour cream
- Salt
- Freshly ground black pepper
- 2 eggs, beaten
- ⅓ cup half-and-half
- 3 cups leftover pulled pork (preferably smoked)

Directions:

1. Supply your smoker with wood pellets and follow the manufacturer's specific start-up procedure. Preheat, with the lid closed, to 350°F.

Braised Short Ribs

Servings: 2 To 4
Cooking Time: 4 Hours

Ingredients:

- 4 beef short ribs
- Salt
- Freshly ground black pepper
- ½ cup beef broth

Directions:

1. Supply your with wood pellets and follow the start-up procedure. Preheat the grill, with the lid closed, to 180°F.
2. Season the ribs on both sides with salt and pepper.
3. Place the ribs directly on the grill grate and smoke for 3 hours.
4. Pull the ribs from the grill and place them on enough aluminum foil to wrap them completely.
5. Increase the grill's temperature to 375°F.
6. Fold in three sides of the foil around the ribs and add the beef broth. Fold in the last side, completely enclosing the ribs and liquid. Return the wrapped ribs to the grill and cook for 45 minutes more. Remove the short ribs from the grill, unwrap them, and serve immediately.

Wood Pellet Grill Pork Crown Roast

Servings: 5
Cooking Time: 1 Hour
Ingredients:
- 13 ribs pork
- 1/4 cup favorite rub
- 1 cup apple juice
- 1 cup Apricot BBQ sauce

Directions:
1. Set the wood pellet temperature to 375°F to preheat for 15 minutes with the lid closed.
2. Meanwhile, season the pork with the rub then let sit for 30 minutes.
3. Wrap the tips of each crown roast with foil to prevent the borns from turning black.
4. Place the meat on the grill grate and cook for 90 minutes. Spray apple juice every 30 minutes.
5. When the meat has reached an internal temperature of 125°F remove the foils.
6. Spray the roast with apple juice again and let cook until the internal temperature has reached 135°F.
7. In the last 10 minutes of cooking, baste the roast with BBQ sauce.
8. Remove from the grill and wrap with foil. Let rest for 15 minutes before serving. Enjoy.

Nutrition Info: Calories 240, Total fat 16g, Saturated fat 6g, Total Carbs 0g, Net Carbs 0g, Protein 23g, Sugar 0g, Fiber 0g, Sodium: 50mg

Smoked Longhorn Cowboy Tri-tip

Servings: 7
Cooking Time: 4 Hours
Ingredients:
- 3 lb tri-tip roast
- 1/8 cup coffee, ground
- 1/4 cup beef rub

Directions:
1. Preheat the grill to 180°F with the lid closed for 15 minutes.
2. Meanwhile, rub the roast with coffee and beef rub. Place the roast on the grill grate and smoke for 3 hours.
3. Remove the roast from the grill and double wrap it with foil. Increase the temperature to 275°F.

4. Return the meat to the grill and let cook for 90 minutes or until the internal temperature reaches 135°F.
5. Remove from the grill, unwrap it and let rest for 10 minutes before serving.
6. Enjoy.

Nutrition Info: Calories 245, Total fat 14g, Saturated fat 4g, Total Carbs 0g, Net Carbs 0g, Protein 23g, Sugar 0g, Fiber 0g, Sodium: 80mg

Smoked Pork Ribs

Servings: 4
Cooking Time: 10 Hours
Ingredients:
- 2 racks back ribs
- 1 cup homemade bbq rub
- 2 12-oz hard apple cider
- 1 cup dark brown sugar
- 2 batches homemade BBQ sauce

Directions:
1. Turn the to smoke setting and remove any membrane from the meat.
2. Place the pork in the and smoke for 5 hours or until it reaches an internal temperature of 175.
3. Increase the grill temperature to 225F. Transfer the meat to a pan sprayed with cooking spray.
4. Pour one bottle of hard apple cider to the pan and rub the brown sugar on top of the ribs.
5. Cover the pan with tin foil and place it back to the Traeger. Cook for 4 hours.
6. Remove the tin foil, increase the temperature to 300F, and place the ribs on the grill grates.
7. Cook for 1 hour brushing the ribs with BBQ sauce 3 times.
8. The ribs should now be falling off the bone. Let rest for 5 minutes before serving.

Nutrition Info: Calories 1073, Total fat 42g, Saturated fat 15g, Total carbs 111g, Net carbs 109g Protein 61g, Sugars 99g, Fiber 3g, Sodium 1663mg

Rosemary Lamb

Servings: 2
Cooking Time: 3 Hours
Ingredients:

- 1 rack of lamb rib, membrane removed
- 12 baby potatoes
- 1 bunch of asparagus, ends trimmed
- Ground black pepper, as needed
- Salt, as needed
- 1 teaspoon dried rosemary
- 2 tablespoons olive oil
- 1/2 cup butter, unsalted

Directions:

1. Switch on the grill, fill the grill hopper with flavored wood pellets, power the grill on by using the control panel, select 'smoke' on the temperature dial, or set the temperature to 225 degrees F and let it preheat for a minimum of 5 minutes.
2. Meanwhile, drizzle oil on both sides of lamb ribs and then sprinkle with rosemary.
3. Take a deep baking dish, place potatoes in it, add butter and mix until coated.
4. When the grill has preheated, open the lid, place lamb ribs on the grill grate along with potatoes in the baking dish, shut the grill and smoke for 3 hours until the internal temperature reaches 145 degrees F.
5. Add asparagus into the baking dish in the last 20 minutes and, when done, remove baking dish from the grill and transfer lamb to a cutting board.
6. Let lamb rest for 15 minutes, cut it into slices, and then serve with potatoes and asparagus.

Nutrition Info: Calories: 355 Cal ;Fat: 12.5 g ;Carbs: 25 g ;Protein: 35 g ;Fiber: 6 g

Stuffed Peppers

Servings: 6
Cooking Time: 5 Minutes
Ingredients:

- 3 bell peppers, sliced in halves
- 1 pound ground beef, lean
- 1 onion, chopped
- 1/2 tbsp red pepper flakes
- 1/2 tbsp salt
- 1/4 tbsp pepper
- 1/2 tbsp garlic powder
- 1/2 tbsp onion powder
- 1/2 cup white rice
- 15 oz stewed tomatoes
- 8 oz tomato sauce

- 6 cups cabbage, shredded
- 1-1/2 cup water
- 2 cups cheddar cheese

Directions:

1. Arrange the pepper halves on a baking tray and set aside.
2. Preheat your grill to 325F.
3. Brown the meat in a large skillet. Add onions, pepper flakes, salt, pepper garlic, and onion and cook until the meat is well cooked.
4. Add rice, stewed tomatoes, tomato sauce, cabbage, and water. Cover and simmer until the rice is well cooked, the cabbage is tender and there is no water in the rice.
5. Place the cooked beef mixture in the pepper halves and top with cheese.
6. Place in the grill and cook for 30 minutes.
7. Serve immediately and enjoy it.

Nutrition Info: Calories: 422 Cal Fat: 22 g Carbohydrates: 24 g   Protein: 34 g Fiber: 5 g

Braised Mediterranean Beef Brisket

Servings: 16
Cooking Time: 5 Hours
Ingredients:

- 3 tablespoons dried rosemary
- .2 tablespoons cumin seeds, ground
- 2 tablespoons dried coriander
- 1 tablespoon dried oregano
- 2 teaspoons ground cinnamon
- ½ teaspoon salt
- 8 pounds beef brisket, sliced into chunks
- 1 cup beef stock

Directions:

1. Mix the rosemary, cumin, coriander, oregano, cinnamon, and salt in a bowl.
2. Massage the spice mix into the beef brisket and allow to rest in the fridge for 12 hours.
3. When ready to cook, fire the Grill to 180F. Use desired wood pellets when cooking. Close the lid and preheat for 15 minutes.
4. Place the brisket fat side down on the grill grate and cook for 4 hours.
5. After 4 hours, turn up the heat to 250F.

6. Continue cooking the beef brisket until the internal temperature reaches 160F. Remove and place on a foil. Crimp the edges of the foil to create a sleeve. Pour in the beef stock.

7. Return the brisket in the foil sleeve and continue cooking for another hour.

Nutrition Info: Calories per serving: 453 ; Protein: 33.5g; Carbs: 1g; Fat: 34g Sugar: 0.1g

Greek-style Roast Leg Of Lamb

Servings: 12
Cooking Time: 1 Hour And 30 Minutes
Ingredients:

- 7 pounds leg of lamb, bone-in, fat trimmed
- 2 lemons, juiced
- 8 cloves of garlic, peeled, minced
- Salt as needed
- Ground black pepper as needed
- 1 teaspoon dried oregano
- 1 teaspoon dried rosemary
- 6 tablespoons olive oil

Directions:

1. Make a small cut into the meat of lamb by using a paring knife, then stir together garlic, oregano, and rosemary and stuff this paste into the slits of the lamb meat.

2. Take a roasting pan, place lamb in it, then rub with lemon juice and olive oil, cover with a plastic wrap and let marinate for a minimum of 8 hours in the refrigerator.

3. When ready to cook, switch on the grill, fill the grill hopper with oak flavored wood pellets, power the grill on by using the control panel, select 'smoke' on the temperature dial, or set the temperature to 400 degrees F and let it preheat for a minimum of 15 minutes.

4. Meanwhile, remove the lamb from the refrigerator, bring it to room temperature, uncover it and then season well with salt and black pepper.

5. When the grill has preheated, open the lid, place food on the grill grate, shut the grill, and smoke for 30 minutes.

6. Change the smoking temperature to 350 degrees F and then continue smoking for 1 hour until the internal temperature reaches 140 degrees F.

7. When done, transfer lamb to a cutting board, let it rest for 15 minutes, then cut it into slices and serve.

Nutrition Info: Calories: 168 Cal ;Fat: 10 g ;Carbs: 2 g ;Protein: 17 g ;Fiber: 0.7 g

Chili Rib Eye Steaks

Servings: 4
Cooking Time: 1 Hour
Ingredients:

- 4 rib-eye steaks, each about 12 ounces
- For the Rub:
- 1 tablespoon minced garlic
- 1 teaspoon salt
- 1 teaspoon brown sugar
- 2 tablespoons red chili powder
- 1 teaspoon ground cumin
- 2 tablespoons Worcestershire sauce
- 2 tablespoons olive oil

Directions:

1. Prepare the rub and for this, take a small bowl, place all of its ingredients in it and then stir until mixed.

2. Brush the paste on all sides of the steak, rub well, then place steaks into a plastic bag and let it marinate for a minimum of 4 hours.

3. When ready to cook, switch on the grill, fill the grill hopper with mesquite flavored wood pellets, power the grill on by using the control panel, select 'smoke' on the temperature dial, or set the temperature to 225 degrees F and let it preheat for a minimum of 15 minutes.

4. When the grill has preheated, open the lid, place steaks on the grill grate, shut the grill, and smoke for 45 minutes until internal temperature reaches 120 degrees F.

5. When done, transfer steaks to a dish, let rest for 15 minutes, and meanwhile, change the smoking temperature of the grill to 450 degrees F and let it preheat for a minimum of 10 minutes.

6. Then return steaks to the grill grate and cook for 3 minutes per side until the internal temperature reaches 140 degrees F.

7. Transfer steaks to a dish, let rest for 5 minutes and then serve.

Nutrition Info: Calories: 293 Cal ;Fat: 0 g ;Carbs: 0 g ;Protein: 32 g ;Fiber: 0 g

Santa Maria Tri-tip

Servings: 4

Cooking Time: 45 Minutes To 1 Hour

Ingredients:

- 2 teaspoons sea salt
- 2 teaspoons freshly ground black pepper
- 2 teaspoons onion powder
- 2 teaspoons garlic powder
- 2 teaspoons dried oregano
- 1 teaspoon cayenne pepper
- 1 teaspoon ground sage
- 1 teaspoon finely chopped fresh rosemary
- 1 (1½ – to 2-pound) tri-tip bottom sirloin

Directions:

1. Supply your with wood pellets and follow the start-up procedure. Preheat the grill, with the lid closed, to 425°F.
2. In a small bowl, combine the salt, pepper, onion powder, garlic powder, oregano, cayenne pepper, sage, and rosemary to create a rub.
3. Season the meat all over with the rub and lay it directly on the grill.
4. Close the lid and smoke for 45 minutes to 1 hour, or until a meat thermometer inserted in the thickest part of the meat reads 120°F for rare, 130°F for medium-rare, or 140°F for medium, keeping in mind that the meat will come up in temperature by about another 5°F during the rest period.
5. Remove the tri-tip from the heat, tent with aluminum foil, and let rest for 15 minutes before slicing against the grain.

FISH AND SEAFOOD RECIPES

Sriracha Salmon

Servings: 4
Cooking Time: 25 Minutes
Ingredients:
- 3-pound salmon, skin on
- For the Marinade:
- 1 teaspoon lime zest
- 1 tablespoon minced garlic
- 1 tablespoon grated ginger
- Sea salt as needed
- Ground black pepper as needed
- 1/4 cup maple syrup
- 2 tablespoons soy sauce
- 2 tablespoons Sriracha sauce
- 1 tablespoon toasted sesame oil
- 1 tablespoon rice vinegar
- 1 teaspoon toasted sesame seeds

Directions:
1. Prepare the marinade and for this, take a small bowl, place all of its ingredients in it, stir until well combined, and then pour the mixture into a large plastic bag.
2. Add salmon in the bag, seal it, turn it upside down to coat salmon with the marinade and let it marinate for a minimum of 2 hours in the refrigerator.
3. When ready to cook, switch on the grill, fill the grill hopper with flavored wood pellets, power the grill on by using the control panel, select 'smoke' on the temperature dial, or set the temperature to 450 degrees F and let it preheat for a minimum of 5 minutes.
4. Meanwhile, take a large baking sheet, line it with parchment paper, place salmon on it skin-side down and then brush with the marinade.
5. When the grill has preheated, open the lid, place baking sheet containing salmon on the grill grate, shut the grill and smoke for 25 minutes until thoroughly cooked.
6. When done, transfer salmon to a dish and then serve.

Nutrition Info: Calories: 360 Cal ;Fat: 21 g ;Carbs: 28 g ;Protein: 16 g ;Fiber: 1.5 g

Lobster Tail

Servings: 2
Cooking Time: 25 Minutes
Ingredients:
- 2 lobster tails
- Salt
- Freshly ground black pepper
- 1 batch Lemon Butter Mop for Seafood

Directions:
1. Supply your smoker with wood pellets and follow the manufacturer's specific start-up procedure. Preheat the grill, with the lid closed, to 375°F.
2. Using kitchen shears, slit the top of the lobster shells, through the center, nearly to the tail. Once cut, expose as much meat as you can through the cut shell.
3. Season the lobster tails all over with salt and pepper.
4. Place the tails directly on the grill grate and grill until their internal temperature reaches 145°F. Remove the lobster from the grill and serve with the mop on the side for dipping.

Togarashi Smoked Salmon

Servings: 10
Cooking Time: 20 Hours 15 Minutes
Ingredients:
- Salmon filet - 2 large
- Togarashi for seasoning
- For Brine:
- Brown sugar - 1 cup
- Water - 4 cups
- Kosher salt - ⅓ cup

Directions:
1. Remove all the thorns from the fish filet.
2. Mix all the brine ingredients until the brown sugar is dissolved completely.
3. Put the mix in a big bowl and add the filet to it.
4. Leave the bowl to refrigerate for 16 hours.
5. After 16 hours, remove the salmon from this mix. Wash and dry it.
6. Place the salmon in the refrigerator for another 2-4 hours. (This step is important. DO NOT SKIP IT.)
7. Season your salmon filet with Togarashi.

8. Start the wood pellet grill with the 'smoke' option and place the salmon on it.
9. Smoke for 4 hours.
10. Make sure the temperature does not go above 180 degrees or below 130 degrees.
11. Remove from the grill and serve it warm with a side dish of your choice.
Nutrition Info: Carbohydrates: 19 g Protein: 10 g Fat: 6 g Sodium: 3772 mg Cholesterol: 29 mg

11. Preheat your smoker to 400 degrees Fahrenheit
12. Add your preferred wood Pellets and transfer the fillets to a non-stick grill tray
13. Transfer to your smoker and smoker for 30-45 minutes until the internal temperature reaches 145 degrees Fahrenheit
14. Allow the fish to rest for 5 minutes and enjoy!
Nutrition Info: Calories: 620 Fats: 50g Carbs: 6g Fiber: 1g

Stuffed Shrimp Tilapia

Servings: 5
Cooking Time: 45 Minutes
Ingredients:
- 5 ounces fresh, farmed tilapia fillets
- 2 tablespoons extra virgin olive oil
- 1and ½ teaspoons smoked paprika
- 1and ½ teaspoons Old Bay seasoning
- Shrimp stuffing
- 1pound shrimp, cooked and deveined
- 1tablespoon salted butter
- 1cup red onion, diced
- 1cup Italian bread crumbs
- ½ cup mayonnaise
- 1large egg, beaten
- 2teaspoons fresh parsley, chopped
- 1and ½ teaspoons salt and pepper

Directions:
1. Take a food processor and add shrimp, chop them up
2. Take a skillet and place it over medium-high heat, add butter and allow it to melt
3. Sauté the onions for 3 minutes
4. Add chopped shrimp with cooled Sautéed onion alongside remaining ingredients listed under stuffing ingredients and transfer to a bowl
5. Cover the mixture and allow it to refrigerate for 60 minutes
6. Rub both sides of the fillet with olive oil
7. Spoon 1/3 cup of the stuffing to the fillet
8. Flatten out the stuffing onto the bottom half of the fillet and fold the Tilapia in half
9. Secure with 2 toothpicks
10. Dust each fillet with smoked paprika and Old Bay seasoning

Lobster Tails

Servings: 4
Cooking Time: 35 Minutes
Ingredients:
- 2 lobster tails, each about 10 ounces
- For the Sauce:
- 2 tablespoons chopped parsley
- 1/4 teaspoon garlic salt
- 1 teaspoon paprika
- 1/4 teaspoon ground black pepper
- 1/4 teaspoon old bay seasoning
- 8 tablespoons butter, unsalted
- 2 tablespoons lemon juice

Directions:
1. Switch on the grill, fill the grill hopper with flavored wood pellets, power the grill on by using the control panel, select 'smoke' on the temperature dial, or set the temperature to 450 degrees F and let it preheat for a minimum of 15 minutes.
2. Meanwhile, prepare the sauce and for this, take a small saucepan, place it over medium-low heat, add butter in it and when it melts, add remaining ingredients for the sauce and stir until combined, set aside until required.
3. Prepare the lobster and for this, cut the shell from the middle to the tail by using kitchen shears and then take the meat from the shell, keeping it attached at the base of the crab tail.
4. Then butterfly the crab meat by making a slit down the middle, then place lobster tails on a baking sheet and pour 1 tablespoon of sauce over each lobster tail, reserve the remaining sauce.
5. When the grill has preheated, open the lid, place crab tails on the grill grate, shut the grill and smoke for 30 minutes until opaque.

6. When done, transfer lobster tails to a dish and then serve with the remaining sauce.
Nutrition Info: Calories: 290 Cal ;Fat: 22 g ;Carbs: 1 g ;Protein: 20 g ;Fiber: 0.3 g

Wood Pellet Togarashi Grilled Salmon

Servings: 6
Cooking Time: 20 Minutes
Ingredients:
- 1 salmon fillet
- 1/4 cup olive oil
- 1/2 tbsp kosher salt
- 1 tbsp Togarashi seasoning

Directions:
1. Preheat the wood pellet grill to 400°F.
2. Place the salmon fillet on a non-stick foil sheet with the skin side up.
3. Rub the olive oil on the salmon and sprinkle with salt and togarashi seasoning.
4. Place the salmon on the preheated grill and close the lid. Cook for 20 minutes or until the internal temperature reaches 145°F.
5. Remove from the grill and serve when hot. Enjoy.
Nutrition Info: Calories 119, Total fat 10g, Saturated fat 2g, Total Carbs 0g, Net Carbs 0g, Protein 6g, Sugar 0g, Fiber 0g, Sodium: 720mg

Charleston Crab Cakes With Remoulade

Servings: 4
Cooking Time: 45 Minutes
Ingredients:
- 1¼ cups mayonnaise
- ¼ cup yellow mustard
- 2 tablespoons sweet pickle relish, with its juices
- 1 tablespoon smoked paprika
- 2 teaspoons Cajun seasoning
- 2 teaspoons prepared horseradish
- 1 teaspoon hot sauce
- 1 garlic clove, finely minced
- 2 pounds fresh lump crabmeat, picked clean
- 20 butter crackers (such as Ritz brand), crushed
- 2 tablespoons Dijon mustard
- 1 cup mayonnaise
- 2 tablespoons freshly squeezed lemon juice
- 1 tablespoon salted butter, melted
- 1 tablespoon Worcestershire sauce
- 1 tablespoon Old Bay seasoning
- 2 teaspoons chopped fresh parsley
- 1 teaspoon ground mustard
- 2 eggs, beaten
- ¼ cup extra-virgin olive oil, divided

Directions:
1. For the remoulade:
2. In a small bowl, combine the mayonnaise, mustard, pickle relish, paprika, Cajun seasoning, horseradish, hot sauce, and garlic.
3. Refrigerate until ready to serve.
4. For the crab cakes:
5. Supply your smoker with wood pellets and follow the manufacturer's specific start-up procedure. Preheat, with the lid closed, to 375°F.
6. Spread the crabmeat on a foil-lined baking sheet and place over indirect heat on the grill, with the lid closed, for 30 minutes.
7. Remove from the heat and let cool for 15 minutes.
8. While the crab cools, combine the crushed crackers, Dijon mustard, mayonnaise, lemon juice, melted butter, Worcestershire sauce, Old Bay, parsley, ground mustard, and eggs until well incorporated.
9. Fold in the smoked crabmeat, then shape the mixture into 8 (1-inch-thick) crab cakes.
10. In a large skillet or cast-iron pan on the grill, heat 2 tablespoons of olive oil. Add half of the crab cakes, close the lid, and smoke for 4 to 5 minutes on each side, or until crispy and golden brown.
11. Remove the crab cakes from the pan and transfer to a wire rack to drain. Pat them to remove any excess oil.
12. Repeat steps 6 and 7 with the remaining oil and crab cakes.
13. Serve the crab cakes with the remoulade.

Dijon-smoked Halibut

Servings: 6
Cooking Time: 2 Hours
Ingredients:

- 4 (6-ounce) halibut steaks
- ¼ cup extra-virgin olive oil
- 2 teaspoons kosher salt
- 1 teaspoon freshly ground black pepper
- ½ cup mayonnaise
- ½ cup sweet pickle relish
- ¼ cup finely chopped sweet onion
- ¼ cup chopped roasted red pepper
- ¼ cup finely chopped tomato
- ¼ cup finely chopped cucumber
- 2 tablespoons Dijon mustard
- 1 teaspoon minced garlic

Directions:
1. Rub the halibut steaks with the olive oil and season on both sides with the salt and pepper. Transfer to a plate, cover with plastic wrap, and refrigerate for 4 hours.
2. Supply your smoker with wood pellets and follow the manufacturer's specific start-up procedure. Preheat, with the lid closed, to 200°F.
3. Remove the halibut from the refrigerator and rub with the mayonnaise.
4. Put the fish directly on the grill grate, close the lid, and smoke for 2 hours, or until opaque and an instant-read thermometer inserted in the fish reads 140°F.
5. While the fish is smoking, combine the pickle relish, onion, roasted red pepper, tomato, cucumber, Dijon mustard, and garlic in a medium bowl. Refrigerate the mustard relish until ready to serve.
6. Serve the halibut steaks hot with the mustard relish.

Citrus Salmon

Servings: 6
Cooking Time: 30 Minutes
Ingredients:
- 2 (1-lb.) salmon fillets
- Salt and freshly ground black pepper, to taste
- 1 tbsp. seafood seasoning
- 2 lemons, sliced
- 2 limes, sliced

Directions:
1. Set the temperature of Grill to 225 degrees F and preheat with closed lid for 15 minutes.

2. Season the salmon fillets with salt, black pepper and seafood seasoning evenly.
3. Place the salmon fillets onto the grill and top each with lemon and lime slices evenly.
4. Cook for about 30 minutes.
5. Remove the salmon fillets from grill and serve hot.

Nutrition Info: Calories per serving: 327; Carbohydrates: 1g; Protein: 36.1g; Fat: 19.8g; Sugar: 0.2g; Sodium: 237mg; Fiber: 0.3g

Bacon-wrapped Shrimp

Servings: 12
Cooking Time: 10 Minutes
Ingredients:
- 1 lb raw shrimp
- 1/2 tbsp salt
- 1/4 tbsp garlic powder
- 1 lb bacon, cut into halves

Directions:
1. Preheat your to 350F.
2. Remove the shells and tails from the shrimp then pat them dry with the paper towels.
3. Sprinkle salt and garlic on the shrimp then wrap with bacon and secure with a toothpick.
4. Place the shrimps on a baking rack greased with cooking spray.
5. Cook for 10 minutes, flip and cook for another 10 minutes or until the bacon is crisp enough.
6. Remove from the and serve.

Nutrition Info: Calories 204, Total fat 14g, Saturated fat 5g, Total carbs 1g, Net carbs 1g Protein 18g, Sugars 0g, Fiber 0g, Sodium 939mg

Juicy Smoked Salmon

Servings: 5
Cooking Time: 50 Minutes
Ingredients:
- ½ cup of sugar
- 2 tablespoon salt
- 2 tablespoons crushed red pepper flakes
- ½ cup fresh mint leaves, chopped
- ¼ cup brandy
- 1(4 pounds) salmon, bones removed

- 2cups alder wood pellets, soaked in water

Directions:

1. Take a medium-sized bowl and add brown sugar, crushed red pepper flakes, mint leaves, salt, and brandy until a paste forms
2. Rub the paste all over your salmon and wrap the salmon with a plastic wrap
3. Allow them to chill overnight
4. Preheat your smoker to 220 degrees Fahrenheit and add wood Pellets
5. Transfer the salmon to the smoker rack and cook smoke for 45 minutes
6. Once the salmon has turned red-brown and the flesh flakes off easily, take it out and serve!

Nutrition Info: Calories: 370 Fats: 28g Carbs: 1g Fiber: 0g

Smoked Shrimp

Servings: 4
Cooking Time: 10 Minutes
Ingredients:

- 4 tablespoons olive oil
- 1 tablespoon Cajun seasoning
- 2 cloves garlic, minced
- 1 tablespoon lemon juice
- Salt to taste
- 2 lb. shrimp, peeled and deveined

Directions:

1. Combine all the ingredients in a sealable plastic bag.
2. Toss to coat evenly.
3. Marinate in the refrigerator for 4 hours.
4. Set the wood pellet grill to high.
5. Preheat it for 15 minutes while the lid is closed.
6. Thread shrimp onto skewers.
7. Grill for 4 minutes per side.
8. Tips: Soak skewers first in water if you are using wooden skewers.

Grilled Blackened Salmon

Servings: 4
Cooking Time: 30 Minutes
Ingredients:

- 4 salmon fillet

- Blackened dry rub
- Italian seasoning powder

Directions:

1. Season salmon fillets with dry rub and seasoning powder.
2. Grill in the wood pellet grill at 325 degrees F for 10 to 15 minutes per side.
3. Tips: You can also drizzle salmon with lemon juice

Lemon Garlic Scallops

Servings: 6
Cooking Time: 5 Minutes
Ingredients:

- 1 dozen scallops
- 2 tablespoons chopped parsley
- Salt as needed
- 1 tablespoon olive oil
- 1 tablespoon butter, unsalted
- 1 teaspoon lemon zest
- For the Garlic Butter:
- ½ teaspoon minced garlic
- 1 lemon, juiced
- 4 tablespoons butter, unsalted, melted

Directions:

1. Switch on the grill, fill the grill hopper with alder flavored wood pellets, power the grill on by using the control panel, select 'smoke' on the temperature dial, or set the temperature to 400 degrees F and let it preheat for a minimum of 15 minutes.
2. Meanwhile, remove frill from scallops, pat dry with paper towels and then season with salt and black pepper.
3. When the grill has preheated, open the lid, place a skillet on the grill grate, add butter and oil, and when the butter melts, place seasoned scallops on it and then cook for 2 minutes until seared.
4. Meanwhile, prepare the garlic butter and for this, take a small bowl, place all of its ingredients in it and then whisk until combined.
5. Flip the scallops, top with some of the prepared garlic butter, and cook for another minute.
6. When done, transfer scallops to a dish, top with remaining garlic butter, sprinkle with parsley and lemon zest, and then serve.

Nutrition Info: Calories: 184 Cal ;Fat: 10 g ;Carbs: 1 g ;Protein: 22 g ;Fiber: 0.2 g

Pacific Northwest Salmon

Servings: 4
Cooking Time: 1 Hour, 15 Minutes
Ingredients:
- 1 (2-pound) half salmon fillet
- 1 batch Dill Seafood Rub
- 2 tablespoons butter, cut into 3 or 4 slices

Directions:
1. Supply your smoker with wood pellets and follow the manufacturer's specific start-up procedure. Preheat the grill, with the lid closed, to 180°F.
2. Season the salmon all over with the rub. Using your hands, work the rub into the flesh.
3. Place the salmon directly on the grill grate, skin-side down, and smoke for 1 hour.
4. Place the butter slices on the salmon, equally spaced. Increase the grill's temperature to 300°F and continue to cook until the salmon's internal temperature reaches 145°F. Remove the salmon from the grill and serve immediately.

Grilled Shrimp Kabobs

Servings: 4
Cooking Time: 10 Minutes
Ingredients:
- 1 lb. colossal shrimp, peeled and deveined
- 2 tbsp. oil
- 1/2 tbsp. garlic salt
- 1/2 tbsp. salt
- 1/8 tbsp. pepper
- 6 skewers

Directions:
1. Preheat your to 375F.
2. Pat the shrimp dry with a paper towel.
3. In a mixing bowl, mix oil, garlic salt, salt, and pepper
4. Toss the shrimp in the mixture until well coated.
5. Skewer the shrimps and cook in the with the lid closed for 4 minutes.

6. Open the lid, flip the skewers and cook for another 4 minutes or until the shrimp is pink and the flesh is opaque.
7. Serve.
Nutrition Info: Calories 325, Total fat 0g, Saturated fat 0g, Total carbs 0g, Net carbs 0g Protein 20g, Sugars 0g, Fiber 0g, Sodium 120mg

Oysters In The Shell

Servings: 4
Cooking Time: 20 Minutes
Ingredients:
- 8 medium oysters, unopened, in the shell, rinsed and scrubbed
- 1 batch Lemon Butter Mop for Seafood

Directions:
1. Supply your smoker with wood pellets and follow the manufacturer's specific start-up procedure. Preheat the grill, with the lid closed, to 375°F.
2. Place the unopened oysters directly on the grill grate and grill for about 20 minutes, or until the oysters are done and their shells open.
3. Discard any oysters that do not open. Shuck the remaining oysters, transfer them to a bowl, and add the mop. Serve immediately.

Super-tasty Trout

Servings: 8
Cooking Time: 5 Hours
Ingredients:
- 1 (7-lb.) whole lake trout, butterflied
- ½ C. kosher salt
- ½ C. fresh rosemary, chopped
- 2 tsp. lemon zest, grated finely

Directions:
1. Rub the trout with salt generously and then, sprinkle with rosemary and lemon zest.
2. Arrange the trout in a large baking dish and refrigerate for about 7-8 hours.
3. Remove the trout from baking dish and rinse under cold running water to remove the salt.
4. With paper towels, pat dry the trout completely.
5. Arrange a wire rack in a sheet pan.

6. Place the trout onto the wire rack, skin side down and refrigerate for about 24 hours.

7. Set the temperature of Grill to 180 degrees F and preheat with closed lid for 15 minutes, using charcoal.

8. Place the trout onto the grill and cook for about 2-4 hours or until desired doneness.

9. Remove the trout from grill and place onto a cutting board for about 5 minutes before serving.

Nutrition Info: Calories per serving: 633; Carbohydrates: 2.4g; Protein: 85.2g; Fat: 31.8g; Sugar: 0g; Sodium: 5000mg; Fiber: 1.6g

Flavor-bursting Prawn Skewers

Servings: 5
Cooking Time: 8 Minutes
Ingredients:
- ¼ C. fresh parsley leaves, minced
- 1 tbsp. garlic, crushed
- 2½ tbsp. olive oil
- 2 tbsp. Thai chili sauce
- 1 tbsp. fresh lime juice
- 1½ pounds prawns, peeled and deveined

Directions:
1. In a large bowl, add all ingredients except for prawns and mix well.
2. In a resealable plastic bag, add marinade and prawns.
3. Seal the bag and shake to coat well
4. Refrigerate for about 20-30 minutes.
5. Set the temperature of Grill to 450 degrees F and preheat with closed lid for 15 minutes.
6. Remove the prawns from marinade and thread onto metal skewers.
7. Arrange the skewers onto the grill and cook for about 4 minutes per side.
8. Remove the skewers from grill and serve hot.

Nutrition Info: Calories per serving: 234; Carbohydrates: 4.9g; Protein: 31.2g; Fat: 9.3g; Sugar: 1.7g; Sodium: 562mg; Fiber: 0.1g

Grilled Tilapia

Servings: 6
Cooking Time: 2o Minutes

Ingredients:
- 2 tsp dried parsley
- ½ tsp garlic powder
- 1 tsp cayenne pepper
- ½ tsp ground black pepper
- ½ tsp thyme
- ½ tsp dried basil
- ½ tsp oregano
- 3 tbsp olive oil
- ½ tsp lemon pepper
- 1 tsp kosher salt
- 1 lemon (juiced)
- 6 tilapia fillets
- 1 ½ tsp creole seafood seasoning

Directions:
1. In a mixing bowl, combine spices
2. Brush the fillets with oil and lemon juice.
3. Liberally, season all sides of the tilapia fillets with the seasoning mix.
4. Preheat your grill to 325°F
5. Place a non-stick BBQ grilling try on the grill and arrange the tilapia fillets onto it.
6. Grill for 15 to 20 minutes
7. Remove fillets and cool down

Nutrition Info: Calories: 176 Cal Fat: 9.6 g Carbohydrates: 1.5 g   Protein: 22.3 g Fiber: 0.5 g

Cajun-blackened Shrimp

Servings: 4
Cooking Time: 20 Minutes
Ingredients:
- 1 pound peeled and deveined shrimp, with tails on
- 1 batch Cajun Rub
- 8 tablespoons (1 stick) butter
- ¼ cup Worcestershire sauce

Directions:
1. Supply your smoker with wood pellets and follow the manufacturer's specific start-up procedure. Preheat the grill, with the lid closed, to 450°F and place a cast-iron skillet on the grill grate. Wait about 10 minutes after your grill has reached temperature, allowing the skillet to get hot.
2. Meanwhile, season the shrimp all over with the rub.

3. When the skillet is hot, place the butter in it to melt. Once the butter melts, stir in the Worcestershire sauce.

4. Add the shrimp and gently stir to coat. Smoke-braise the shrimp for about 10 minutes per side, until opaque and cooked through. Remove the shrimp from the grill and serve immediately.

Grilled Shrimp Scampi

Servings: 4
Cooking Time: 10 Minutes
Ingredients:
- 1 lb raw shrimp, tail on
- 1/2 cup salted butter, melted
- 1/4 cup white wine, dry
- 1/2 tbsp fresh garlic, chopped
- 1 tbsp lemon juice
- 1/2 tbsp garlic powder
- 1/2 tbsp salt

Directions:
1. Preheat your wood pellet grill to 400°F with a cast iron inside.
2. In a mixing bowl, mix butter, wine, garlic, and juice then pour in the cast iron. Let the mixture mix for 4 minutes.
3. Sprinkle garlic and salt on the shrimp then place it on the cast iron. Grill for 10 minutes with the lid closed.
4. Remove the shrimp from the grill and serve when hot. Enjoy.
Nutrition Info: Calories 298, Total fat 24g, Saturated fat 15g, Total Carbs 2g, Net Carbs 2g, Protein 16g, Sugar 0g, Fiber 0g, Sodium: 1091mg, Potassium 389mg

Wood Pellet Salt And Pepper Spot Prawn Skewers

Servings: 6
Cooking Time: 10 Minutes
Ingredients:
- 2 lb spot prawns, clean
- 2 tbsp oil
- Salt and pepper to taste

Directions:

1. Preheat your grill to 400°F.
2. Meanwhile, soak the skewers then skewer with the prawns.
3. Brush with oil then season with salt and pepper to taste.
4. Place the skewers in the grill, close the lid, and cook for 5 minutes on each side.
5. Remove from the grill and serve. Enjoy.
Nutrition Info: Calories 221, Total fat 7g, Saturated fat 1g, Total Carbs 2g, Net Carbs 2g, Protein 34g, Sugar 0g, Fiber 0g, Sodium: 1481mg, Potassium 239mg

Wine Infused Salmon

Servings: 4
Cooking Time: 5 Hours
Ingredients:
- 2 C. low-sodium soy sauce
- 1 C. dry white wine
- 1 C. water
- ½ tsp. Tabasco sauce
- 1/3 C. sugar
- ¼ C. salt
- ½ tsp. garlic powder
- ½ tsp. onion powder
- Freshly ground black pepper, to taste
- 4 (6-oz.) salmon fillets

Directions:
1. In a large bowl, add all ingredients except salmon and stir until sugar is dissolved.
2. Add salmon fillets and coat with brine well.
3. Refrigerate, covered overnight.
4. Remove salmon from bowl and rinse under cold running water.
5. With paper towels, pat dry the salmon fillets.
6. Arrange a wire rack in a sheet pan.
7. Place the salmon fillets onto wire rack, skin side down and set aside to cool for about 1 hour.
8. Set the temperature of Grill to 165 degrees F and preheat with closed lid for 15 minutes, using charcoal.
9. Place the salmon fillets onto the grill, skin side down and cook for about 3-5 hours or until desired doneness.

10. Remove the salmon fillets from grill and serve hot.
Nutrition Info: Calories per serving: 377; Carbohydrates: 26.3g; Protein: 41.1g; Fat: 10.5g; Sugar: 25.1g; Sodium: 14000mg; Fiber: 0g

Lively Flavored Shrimp

Servings: 6
Cooking Time: 30 Minutes
Ingredients:
- 8 oz. salted butter, melted
- ¼ C. Worcestershire sauce
- ¼ C. fresh parsley, chopped
- 1 lemon, quartered
- 2 lb. jumbo shrimp, peeled and deveined
- 3 tbsp. BBQ rub

Directions:
1. In a metal baking pan, add all ingredients except for shrimp and BBQ rub and mix well.
2. Season the shrimp with BBQ rub evenly.
3. Add the shrimp in the pan with butter mixture and coat well.
4. Set aside for about 20-30 minutes.
5. Set the temperature of Grill to 250 degrees F and preheat with closed lid for 15 minutes.
6. Place the pan onto the grill and cook for about 25-30 minutes.
7. Remove the pan from grill and serve hot.
Nutrition Info: Calories per serving: 462; Carbohydrates: 4.7g; Protein: 34.9g; Fat: 33.3g; Sugar: 2.1g; Sodium: 485mg; Fiber: 0.2g

Grilled Lingcod

Servings: 6
Cooking Time: 15 Minutes
Ingredients:
- 2 lb lingcod fillets
- 1/2 tbsp salt
- 1/2 tbsp white pepper
- 1/4 tbsp cayenne pepper
- Lemon wedges

Directions:
1. Preheat your to 375F.

2. Place the lingcod on a parchment paper or on a grill mat
3. Season the fish with salt, pepper, and top with lemon wedges.
4. Cook the fish for 15 minutes or until the internal temperature reaches 145F.
Nutrition Info: Calories 245, Total fat 2g, Saturated fat 0g, Total carbs 2g, Net carbs 0g Protein 52g, Sugars 1g, Fiber 1g, Sodium 442mg

Lobster Tail

Servings: 2
Cooking Time: 15 Minutes
Ingredients:
- 10 oz lobster tail
- 1/4 tbsp old bay seasoning
- 1/4 tbsp Himalayan salt
- 2 tbsp butter, melted
- 1 tbsp fresh parsley, chopped

Directions:
1. Preheat your to 450F.
2. Slice the tail down the middle then season it with bay seasoning and salt.
3. Place the tails directly on the grill with the meat side down. Grill for 15 minutes or until the internal temperature reaches 140F.
4. Remove from the and drizzle with butter.
5. Serve when hot garnished with parsley.
Nutrition Info: Calories 305, Total fat 14g, Saturated fat 8g, Total carbs 5g, Net carbs 5g Protein 38g, Sugars 0g, Fiber 0g, Sodium 684mg

Salmon With Togarashi

Servings: 3
Cooking Time: 20 Minutes
Ingredients:
- 1 salmon fillet
- 1/4 cup olive oil
- 1/2 tbsp kosher salt
- 1 tbsp Togarashi seasoning

Directions:
1. Preheat your to 400F.
2. Place the salmon on a sheet lined with non-stick foil with the skin side down.

3. Rub the oil into the meat then sprinkle salt and Togarashi.

4. Place the salmon on the grill and cook for 20 minutes or until the internal temperature reaches 145F with the lid closed.

5. Remove from the and serve when hot.

Nutrition Info: Calories 119, Total fat 10g, Saturated fat 2g, Total carbs 0g, Net carbs 0g Protein 0g, Sugars 0g, Fiber 0g, Sodium 720mg

Bacon-wrapped Scallops

Servings: 4
Cooking Time: 30 Minutes
Ingredients:
- 12 scallops
- 12 bacon slices
- 3 tablespoons lemon juice
- Pepper to taste

Directions:
1. Turn on your wood pellet grill.
2. Set it to smoke.
3. Let it burn for 5 minutes while the lid is open.
4. Set it to 400 degrees F.
5. Wrap the scallops with bacon.
6. Secure with a toothpick.
7. Drizzle with the lemon juice and season with pepper.
8. Add the scallops to a baking tray.
9. Place the tray on the grill.
10. Grill for 20 minutes.
11. Serving Suggestion: Serve with sweet chili sauce.

Nutrition Info: Calories: 180.3 Fat: 8 g Cholesterol: 590.2 mg Carbohydrates: 3 g Fiber: 0 g Sugars: 0 g Protein: 22 g

Cod With Lemon Herb Butter

Servings: 4
Cooking Time: 15 Minutes
Ingredients:
- 4 tablespoons butter
- 1 clove garlic, minced
- 1 tablespoon tarragon, chopped
- 1 tablespoon lemon juice
- 1 teaspoon lemon zest

- Salt and pepper to taste
- 1 lb. cod fillet

Directions:
1. Preheat the wood pellet grill to high for 15 minutes while the lid is closed.
2. In a bowl, mix the butter, garlic, tarragon, lemon juice and lemon zest, salt and pepper.
3. Place the fish in a baking pan.
4. Spread the butter mixture on top.
5. Bake the fish for 15 minutes.
6. Tips: You can also use other white fish fillet for this recipe.

Summer Paella

Servings: 6
Cooking Time: 45 Minutes
Ingredients:
- 6 tablespoons extra-virgin olive oil, divided, plus more for drizzling
- 2 green or red bell peppers, cored, seeded, and diced
- 2 medium onions, diced
- 2 garlic cloves, slivered
- 1 (29-ounce) can tomato purée
- 1½ pounds chicken thighs
- Kosher salt
- 1½ pounds tail-on shrimp, peeled and deveined
- 1 cup dried thinly sliced chorizo sausage
- 1 tablespoon smoked paprika
- 1½ teaspoons saffron threads
- 2 quarts chicken broth
- 3½ cups white rice
- 2 (7½-ounce) cans chipotle chiles in adobo sauce
- 1½ pounds fresh clams, soaked in cold water for 15 to 20 minutes2 tablespoons chopped fresh parsley
- 2 lemons, cut into wedges, for serving

Directions:
1. Make the sofrito: On the stove top, in a saucepan over medium-low heat, combine ¼ cup of olive oil, the bell peppers, onions, and garlic, and cook for 5 minutes, or until the onions are translucent.
2. Stir in the tomato purée, reduce the heat to low, and simmer, stirring frequently, until most of the

liquid has evaporated, about 30 minutes. Set aside. (Note: The sofrito can be made in advance and refrigerated.)

3. Supply your smoker with wood pellets and follow the manufacturer's specific start-up procedure. Preheat, with the lid closed, to 450°F.

4. Heat a large paella pan on the smoker and add the remaining 2 tablespoons of olive oil.

5. Add the chicken thighs, season lightly with salt, and brown for 6 to 10 minutes, then push to the outer edge of the pan.

6. Add the shrimp, season with salt, close the lid, and smoke for 3 minutes.

7. Add the sofrito, chorizo, paprika, and saffron, and stir together.

8. In a separate bowl, combine the chicken broth, uncooked rice, and 1 tablespoon of salt, stirring until well combined.

9. Add the broth-rice mixture to the paella pan, spreading it evenly over the other ingredients.

10. Close the lid and smoke for 5 minutes, then add the chipotle chiles and clams on top of the rice.

11. Close the lid and continue to smoke the paella for about 30 minutes, or until all of the liquid is absorbed.

12. Remove the pan from the grill, cover tightly with aluminum foil, and let rest off the heat for 5 minutes.

13. Drizzle with olive oil, sprinkle with the fresh parsley, and serve with the lemon wedges.

Cider Salmon

Servings: 4
Cooking Time: 1 Hour
Ingredients:
- 1 ½ pound salmon fillet, skin-on, center-cut, pin bone removed
- For the Brine:
- 4 juniper berries, crushed
- 1 bay leaf, crumbled
- 1 piece star anise, broken
- 1 1/2 cups apple cider
- For the Cure:
- 1/2 cup salt
- 1 teaspoon ground black pepper
- 1/4 cup brown sugar

- 2 teaspoons barbecue rub

Directions:

1. Prepare the brine and for this, take a large container, add all of its ingredients in it, stir until mixed, then add salmon and let soak for a minimum of 8 hours in the refrigerator.

2. Meanwhile, prepare the cure and for this, take a small bowl, place all of its ingredients in it and stir until combined.

3. After 8 hours, remove salmon from the brine, then take a baking dish, place half of the cure in it, top with salmon skin-side down, sprinkle remaining cure on top, cover with plastic wrap and let it rest for 1 hour in the refrigerator.

4. When ready to cook, switch on the grill, fill the grill hopper with oak flavored wood pellets, power the grill on by using the control panel, select 'smoke' on the temperature dial, or set the temperature to 200 degrees F and let it preheat for a minimum of 5 minutes.

5. Meanwhile, remove salmon from the cure, pat dry with paper towels, and then sprinkle with black pepper.

6. When the grill has preheated, open the lid, place salmon on the grill grate, shut the grill, and smoke for 1 hour until the internal temperature reaches 150 degrees F.

7. When done, transfer salmon to a cutting board, let it rest for 5 minutes, then remove the skin and serve.

Nutrition Info: Calories: 233 Cal ;Fat: 14 g ;Carbs: 0 g ;Protein: 25 g ;Fiber: 0 g

Wood Pellet Rockfish

Servings: 6
Cooking Time: 20 Minutes
Ingredients:
- 6 rockfish fillets
- 1 lemon, sliced
- 3/4 tbsp Himalayan salt
- 2 tbsp fresh dill, chopped
- 1/2 tbsp garlic powder
- 1/2 tbsp onion powder
- 6 tbsp butter

Directions:

1. Preheat your wood pellet grill to 375°F.
2. Place the rockfish in a baking dish and season with salt, dill, garlic, and onion.
3. Place butter on top of the fish then close the lid. Cook for 20 minutes or until the fish is no longer translucent.
4. Remove from grill and let sit for 5 minutes before serving. enjoy.

Nutrition Info: Calories 270, Total fat 17g, Saturated fat 9g, Total Carbs 2g, Net Carbs 0g, Protein 28g, Sugar 0g, Fiber 0g, Sodium: 381mg

Cajun Catfish

Servings: 6
Cooking Time: 15 Minutes
Ingredients:
- 2½ pounds catfish fillets
- 2 tablespoons olive oil
- 1 batch Cajun Rub

Directions:
1. Supply your smoker with wood pellets and follow the manufacturer's specific start-up procedure. Preheat the grill, with the lid closed, to 300°F.
2. Coat the catfish fillets all over with olive oil and season with the rub. Using your hands, work the rub into the flesh.
3. Place the fillets directly on the grill grate and smoke until their internal temperature reaches 145°F. Remove the catfish from the grill and serve immediately

Grilled King Crab Legs

Servings: 4
Cooking Time: 25 Minutes
Ingredients:
- 4 pounds king crab legs (split)
- 4 tbsp lemon juice
- 2 tbsp garlic powder
- 1 cup butter (melted)
- 2 tsp brown sugar
- 2 tsp paprika
- Black pepper (depends to your liking)

Directions:

1. In a mixing bowl, combine the lemon juice, butter, sugar, garlic, paprika and pepper.
2. Arrange the split crab on a baking sheet, split side up. Drizzle ¾ of the butter mixture over the crab legs. Configure your pellet grill for indirect cooking and preheat it to 225°F, using mesquite wood pellets.
3. Arrange the crab legs onto the grill grate, shell side down. Cover the grill and cook 25 minutes.
4. Remove the crab legs from the grill. Serve and top with the remaining butter mixture.

Nutrition Info: Calories: 480 Cal Fat: 53.2 g Carbohydrates: 6.1 g Protein: 88.6 g Fiber: 1.2 g

No-fuss Tuna Burgers

Servings: 6
Cooking Time: 15 Minutes
Ingredients:
- 2 lb. tuna steak
- 1 green bell pepper, seeded and chopped
- 1 white onion, chopped
- 2 eggs
- 1 tsp. soy sauce
- 1 tbsp. blackened Saskatchewan rub
- Salt and freshly ground black pepper, to taste

Directions:
1. Set the temperature of Grill to 500 degrees F and preheat with closed lid for 15 minutes.
2. In a bowl, add all the ingredients and mix until well combined.
3. With greased hands, make patties from mixture.
4. Place the patties onto the grill close to the edges and cook for about 10-15 minutes, flipping once halfway through.
5. Serve hot.

Nutrition Info: Calories per serving: 313; Carbohydrates: 3.4g; Protein: 47.5g; Fat: 11g; Sugar: 1.9g; Sodium: 174mg; Fiber: 0.7g

Wood Pellet Teriyaki Smoked Shrimp

Servings: 6
Cooking Time: 10 Minutes
Ingredients:
- 1 lb tail-on shrimp, uncooked
- 1/2 tbsp onion powder

- 1/2 tbsp salt
- 1/2 tbsp Garlic powder
- 4 tbsp Teriyaki sauce
- 4 tbsp sriracha mayo
- 2 tbsp green onion, minced

Directions:

1. Peel the shrimps leaving the tails then wash them removing any vein left over. Drain and pat with a paper towel to drain.
2. Preheat the wood pellet to 450°F
3. Season the shrimp with onion, salt, and garlic then place it on the grill to cook for 5 minutes on each side.
4. Remove the shrimp from the grill and toss it with teriyaki sauce. Serve garnished with mayo and onions. Enjoy.

Nutrition Info: Calories 87, Total fat 0g, Saturated fat 0g, Total Carbs 2g, Net Carbs 2g, Protein 16g, Sugar 1g, Fiber 0g, Sodium: 1241mg

Mussels With Pancetta Aïoli

Servings: 4
Cooking Time: 30 Minutes

Ingredients:

- ¾ cup mayonnaise (to make your own, see page 460)
- 1tablespoon minced garlic, or more to taste
- 1.4-ounce slice pancetta, chopped
- Salt and pepper
- 4 pounds mussels
- 8 thick slices Italian bread
- ¼ cup good-quality olive oil

Directions:

1. Whisk the mayonnaise and garlic together in a small bowl. Put the pancetta in a small cold skillet, turn the heat to low; cook, occasionally stir, until most of the fat is rendered and the meat turns golden and crisp about 5 minutes. Drain on a paper towel, then stir into the mayonnaise along with 1 teaspoon of the rendered fat from the pan. Taste and add more garlic and some salt if you like. Cover and refrigerate until you're ready to serve. (You can make the aïoli up to several days ahead; refrigerate in an airtight container.)

2. Start the coals or heat a gas grill for direct hot cooking. Make sure the grates are clean.
3. Rinse the mussels and pull off any beards. Discard any that are broken or don't close when tapped.
4. Brush both sides of the bread slices with the oil. Put the bread on the grill directly over the fire. Close the lid and toast, turning once, until it develops grill marks with some charring, 1 to 2 minutes per side. Remove from the grill and keep warm.
5. Scatter the mussels onto the grill directly over the fire, spreading them out, so they are in a single layer. Immediately close the lid and cook for 3 minutes. Transfer the open mussels to a large bowl with tongs. If any have not opened, leave them on the grill, close the lid, and cook for another minute or 2, checking frequently and removing open mussels until they are all off the grill.
6. Dollop the aïoli over the tops of the mussels and use a large spoon to turn them over to coat them. Serve the mussels drizzled with their juices, either over (or alongside) the bread.

Nutrition Info: Calories: 159 Fats: 6.1 g Cholesterol: 0 mg Carbohydrates: 14.95 g Fiber: 0 g Sugars: 0 g Proteins: 9.57 g

Grilled Lingcod

Servings: 6
Cooking Time: 15 Minutes

Ingredients:

- 2 lb lingcod fillets
- 1/2 tbsp salt
- 1/2 tbsp white pepper
- 1/4 tbsp cayenne
- Lemon wedges

Directions:

1. Preheat the wood pellet grill to 375°F.
2. Place the lingcod on a parchment paper and season it with salt, white pepper, cayenne pepper then top with the lemon.
3. Place the fish on the grill and cook for 15 minutes or until the internal temperature reaches 145°F.
4. Serve and enjoy.

Nutrition Info: Calories 245, Total fat 2g, Saturated fat 0g, Total Carbs 2g, Net Carbs 1g, Protein 52g, Sugar 1g, Fiber 1g, Sodium: 442mg, Potassium 649mg

Smoked Shrimp

Servings: 6
Cooking Time: 10 Minutes
Ingredients:
- 1 lb tail-on shrimp, uncooked
- 1/2 tbsp onion powder
- 1/2 tbsp garlic powder
- 1/2 tbsp salt
- 4 tbsp teriyaki sauce
- 2 tbsp green onion, minced
- 4 tbsp sriracha mayo

Directions:
1. Peel the shrimp shells leaving the tail on then wash well and rise.
2. Drain well and pat dry with a paper towel.
3. Preheat your to 450F.
4. Season the shrimp with onion powder, garlic powder, and salt. Place the shrimp in the and cook for 6 minutes on each side.
5. Remove the shrimp from the and toss with teriyaki sauce then garnish with onions and mayo.

Nutrition Info: Calories 87, Total fat 0g, Saturated fat 0g, Total carbs 2g, Net carbs 2g Protein 16g, Sugars 0g, Fiber 0g, Sodium 1241mg

Salmon With Avocado Salsa

Servings: 6
Cooking Time: 20 Minutes
Ingredients:
- 3 lb. salmon fillet
- Garlic salt and pepper to taste
- 4 cups avocado, sliced into cubes
- 1 onion, chopped
- 1 jalapeño pepper, minced
- 1 tablespoon lime juice
- 1 tablespoon olive oil
- ¼ cup cilantro, chopped
- Salt to taste

Directions:

1. Sprinkle both sides of salmon with garlic salt and pepper.
2. Set the wood pellet grill to smoke.
3. Grill the salmon for 7 to 8 minutes per side.
4. While waiting, prepare the salsa by combining the remaining ingredients in a bowl.
5. Serve salmon with the avocado salsa.
6. Tips: You can also use tomato salsa for this recipe if you don't have avocados.

Crazy Delicious Lobster Tails

Servings: 4
Cooking Time: 25 Minutes
Ingredients:
- ½ C. butter, melted
- 2 garlic cloves, minced
- 2 tsp. fresh lemon juice
- Salt and freshly ground black pepper, to taste
- 4 (8-oz.) lobster tails

Directions:
1. Set the temperature of Grill to 450 degrees F and preheat with closed lid for 15 minutes.
2. In a metal pan, add all ingredients except for lobster tails and mix well.
3. Place the pan onto the grill and cook for about 10 minutes.
4. Meanwhile, cut down the top of the shell and expose lobster meat.
5. Remove pan of butter mixture from grill.
6. Coat the lobster meat with butter mixture.
7. Place the lobster tails onto the grill and cook for about 15 minutes, coating with butter mixture once halfway through.
8. Remove from grill and serve hot.

Nutrition Info: Calories per serving: 409; Carbohydrates: 0.6g; Protein: 43.5g; Fat: 24.9g; Sugar: 0.1g; Sodium: 1305mg; Fiber: 0g

Omega-3 Rich Salmon

Servings: 6
Cooking Time: 20 Minutes
Ingredients:
- 6 (6-oz.) skinless salmon fillets
- 1/3 C. olive oil

- ¼ C. spice rub
- ¼ C. honey
- 2 tbsp. Sriracha
- 2 tbsp. fresh lime juice

Directions:

1. Set the temperature of Grill to 300 degrees F and preheat with closed lid for 15 minutes.
2. Coat salmon fillets with olive oil and season with rub evenly.
3. In a small bowl, mix together remaining ingredients.
4. Arrange salmon fillets onto the grill, flat-side up and cook for about 7-10 minutes per side, coating with honey mixture once halfway through.
5. Serve hot alongside remaining honey mixture.

Nutrition Info: Calories per serving: 384; Carbohydrates: 15.7g; Protein: 33g; Fat: 21.7g; Sugar: 11.6g; Sodium: 621mg; Fiber: 0g

Enticing Mahi-mahi

Servings: 4
Cooking Time: 10 Minutes
Ingredients:

- 4 (6-oz.) mahi-mahi fillets
- 2 tbsp. olive oil
- Salt and freshly ground black pepper, to taste

Directions:

1. Set the temperature of Grill to 350 degrees F and preheat with closed lid for 15 minutes.
2. Coat fish fillets with olive oil and season with salt and black pepper evenly.
3. Place the fish fillets onto the grill and cook for about 5 minutes per side.
4. Remove the fish fillets from grill and serve hot.

Nutrition Info: Calories per serving: 195; Carbohydrates: 0g; Protein: 31.6g; Fat: 7g; Sugar: 0g; Sodium: 182mg; Fiber: 0g

Grilled Tuna

Servings: 4
Cooking Time: 4 Minutes
Ingredients:

- 4 (6 ounce each) tuna steaks (1 inch thick)
- 1 lemon (juiced)

- 1 clove garlic (minced)
- 1 tsp chili
- 2 tbsp extra virgin olive oil
- 1 cup white wine
- 3 tbsp brown sugar
- 1 tsp rosemary

Directions:

1. Combine lemon, chili, white wine, sugar, rosemary, olive oil and garlic. Add the tuna steaks and toss to combine.
2. Transfer the tuna and marinade to a zip-lock bag. Refrigerate for 3 hours.
3. Remove the tuna steaks from the marinade and let them rest for about 1 hour
4. Start your grill on smoke, leaving the lid opened for 5 minutes, or until fire starts.
5. Do not open lid to preheat until 15 minutes to the setting "HIGH"
6. Grease the grill grate with oil and place the tuna on the grill grate. Grill tuna steaks for 4 minutes, 2 minutes per side.
7. Remove the tuna from the grill and let them rest for a few minutes.

Nutrition Info: Calories: 137 Cal Fat: 17.8 g Carbohydrates: 10.2 g Protein: 51.2 g Fiber: 0.6 g

Grilled Salmon

Servings: 4
Cooking Time: 25 Minutes
Ingredients:

- 1 (2-pound) half salmon fillet
- 3 tablespoons mayonnaise
- 1 batch Dill Seafood Rub

Directions:

1. Supply your smoker with wood pellets and follow the manufacturer's specific start-up procedure. Preheat the grill, with the lid closed, to 325°F.
2. Using your hands, rub the salmon fillet all over with the mayonnaise and sprinkle it with the rub.
3. Place the salmon directly on the grill grate, skin-side down, and grill until its internal temperature reaches 145°F. Remove the salmon from the grill and serve immediately.

Fish Fillets With Pesto

Servings: 6
Cooking Time: 15 Minutes
Ingredients:
- 2 cups fresh basil
- 1 cup parsley, chopped
- 1/2 cup walnuts
- 1/2 cup olive oil
- 1 cup Parmesan cheese, grated
- Salt and pepper to taste
- 4 white fish fillets

Directions:
1. Preheat the wood pellet grill to high for 15 minutes while the lid is closed.
2. Add all the ingredients except fish to a food processor.
3. Pulse until smooth. Set aside.
4. Season fish with salt and pepper.
5. Grill for 6 to 7 minutes per side.
6. Serve with the pesto sauce.
7. Tips: You can also spread a little bit of the pesto on the fish before grilling.

Grilled Rainbow Trout

Servings: 6
Cooking Time: 2 Hours
Ingredients:
- 6 rainbow trout, cleaned, butterfly
- For the Brine:
- 1/4 cup salt
- 1 tablespoon ground black pepper
- 1/2 cup brown sugar
- 2 tablespoons soy sauce
- 16 cups water

Directions:
1. Prepare the brine and for this, take a large container, add all of its ingredients in it, stir until sugar has dissolved, then add trout and let soak for 1 hour in the refrigerator.
2. When ready to cook, switch on the grill, fill the grill hopper with oak flavored wood pellets, power the grill on by using the control panel, select 'smoke' on the temperature dial, or set the temperature to 225 degrees F and let it preheat for a minimum of 15 minutes.
3. Meanwhile, remove trout from the brine and pat dry with paper towels.
4. When the grill has preheated, open the lid, place trout on the grill grate, shut the grill and smoke for 2 hours until thoroughly cooked and tender.
5. When done, transfer trout to a dish and then serve.
Nutrition Info: Calories: 250 Cal ;Fat: 12 g ;Carbs: 1.4 g ;Protein: 33 g ;Fiber: 0.3 g

Cajun Seasoned Shrimp

Servings: 4
Cooking Time: 16-20 Minutes
Ingredients:
- 20 pieces of jumbo Shrimp
- 1/2 teaspoon of Cajun seasoning
- 1tablespoon of Canola oil
- 1teaspoon of magic shrimp seasoning

Directions:
1. Take a large bowl and add canola oil, shrimp, and seasonings.
2. Mix well for fine coating.
3. Now put the shrimp on skewers.
4. Put the grill grate inside the grill and set a timer to 8 minutes at high for preheating.
5. Once the grill is preheated, open the unit and place the shrimp skewers inside.
6. Cook the shrimp for 2 minutes.
7. Open the unit to flip the shrimp and cook for another 2 minutes at medium.
8. Own done, serve.
Nutrition Info: Calories: 382 Total Fat: 7.4g Saturated Fat: 0g Cholesterol: 350mg Sodium: 2208mg Total Carbohydrate: 23.9g Dietary Fiber 2.6g Total Sugars: 2.6g Protein: 50.2g

Jerk Shrimp

Servings: 12
Cooking Time: 6 Minutes
Ingredients:
- 2 pounds shrimp, peeled, deveined
- 3 tablespoons olive oil
- For the Spice Mix:
- 1 teaspoon garlic powder

- 1 teaspoon of sea salt
- 1/4 teaspoon ground cayenne
- 1 tablespoon brown sugar
- 1/8 teaspoon smoked paprika
- 1 tablespoon smoked paprika
- 1/4 teaspoon ground thyme
- 1 lime, zested

Directions:

1. Switch on the grill, fill the grill hopper with flavored wood pellets, power the grill on by using the control panel, select 'smoke' on the temperature dial, or set the temperature to 450 degrees F and let it preheat for a minimum of 5 minutes.

2. Meanwhile, prepare the spice mix and for this, take a small bowl, place all of its ingredients in it and stir until mixed.

3. Take a large bowl, place shrimps in it, sprinkle with prepared spice mix, drizzle with oil and toss until well coated.

4. When the grill has preheated, open the lid, place shrimps on the grill grate, shut the grill and smoke for 3 minutes per side until firm and thoroughly cooked.

5. When done, transfer shrimps to a dish and then serve.

Nutrition Info: Calories: 131 Cal ;Fat: 4.3 g ;Carbs: 0 g ;Protein: 22 g ;Fiber: 0 g

Teriyaki Smoked Shrimp

Servings: 6
Cooking Time: 20 Minutes
Ingredients:
- Uncooked shrimp - 1 lb.
- Onion powder - ½ tbsp
- Garlic powder - ½ tbsp
- Teriyaki sauce - 4 tbsp
- Mayo - 4 tbsp
- Minced green onion - 2 tbsp
- Salt - ½ tbsp

Directions:

1. Remove the shells from the shrimp and wash thoroughly.

2. Preheat the wood pellet grill to 450 degrees.

3. Season with garlic powder, onion powder, and salt.

4. Cook the shrimp for 5-6 minutes on each side.

5. Once cooked, remove the shrimp from the grill and garnish it with spring onion, teriyaki sauce, and mayo.

Nutrition Info: Carbohydrates: 2 g Protein: 16 g Sodium: 1241 mg Cholesterol: 190 mg

Wood Pellet Garlic Dill Smoked Salmon

Servings: 12
Cooking Time: 4 Hours
Ingredients:
- 2 salmon fillets
- Brine
- 4 cups water
- 1 cup brown sugar
- 1/3 cup kosher salt
- Seasoning
- 3 tbsp minced garlic
- 1 tbsp fresh dill, chopped

Directions:

1. In a zip lock bag, combine the brine ingredients until all sugar has dissolved. Place the salmon in the bag and refrigerate overnight.

2. Remove the salmon from the brine, rinse with water and pat dry with a paper towel. Let it rest for 2-4 hours at room temperature.

3. Season the salmon with garlic and dill generously.

4. Fire up the wood pellet grill to smoke and place the salmon on a cooling rack that is coated with cooking spray.

5. Place the rack in the smoker and close the lid.

6. Smoke the salmon for 4 hours until the smoke is between 130-180°F.

7. Remove the salmon from the grill and serve with crackers. Enjoy

Nutrition Info: Calories 139, Total fat 5g, Saturated fat 1g, Total Carbs 16g, Net Carbs 16g, Protein 9g, Sugar 0g, Fiber 0g, Sodium: 3143mg

Chilean Sea Bass

Servings: 6
Cooking Time: 40 Minutes
Ingredients:

- 4 sea bass fillets, skinless, each about 6 ounces
- Chicken rub as needed
- 8 tablespoons butter, unsalted
- 2 tablespoons chopped thyme leaves
- Lemon slices for serving
- For the Marinade:
- 1 lemon, juiced
- 4 teaspoons minced garlic
- 1 tablespoon chopped thyme
- 1 teaspoon blackened rub
- 1 tablespoon chopped oregano
- 1/4 cup oil

Directions:

1. Prepare the marinade and for this, take a small bowl, place all of its ingredients in it, stir until well combined, and then pour the mixture into a large plastic bag.
2. Add fillets in the bag, seal it, turn it upside down to coat fillets with the marinade and let it marinate for a minimum of 30 minutes in the refrigerator.
3. When ready to cook, switch on the grill, fill the grill hopper with apple-flavored wood pellets, power the grill on by using the control panel, select 'smoke' on the temperature dial, or set the temperature to 325 degrees F and let it preheat for a minimum of 15 minutes.
4. Meanwhile, take a large baking pan and place butter on it.
5. When the grill has preheated, open the lid, place baking pan on the grill grate, and wait until butter melts.
6. Remove fillets from the marinade, pour marinade into the pan with melted butter, then season fillets with chicken rubs until coated on all sides, then place them into the pan, shut the grill and cook for 30 minutes until internal temperature reaches 160 degrees F, frequently basting with the butter sauce.
7. When done, transfer fillets to a dish, sprinkle with thyme and then serve with lemon slices.

Nutrition Info: Calories: 232 Cal ;Fat: 12.2 g ;Carbs: 0.8 g ;Protein: 28.2 g ;Fiber: 0.1 g

Grilled Shrimp

Servings: 4

Cooking Time: 15 Minutes

Ingredients:
- Jumbo shrimp peeled and cleaned - 1 lb.
- Oil - 2 tbsp
- Salt - ½ tbsp
- Skewers - 4-5
- Pepper - ⅛ tbsp
- Garlic salt - ½ tbsp

Directions:

1. Preheat the wood pellet grill to 375 degrees.
2. Mix all the ingredients in a small bowl.
3. After washing and drying the shrimp, mix it well with the oil and seasonings.
4. Add skewers to the shrimp and set the bowl of shrimp aside.
5. Open the skewers and flip them.
6. Cook for 4 more minutes. Remove when the shrimp is opaque and pink.

Nutrition Info: Carbohydrates: 1.3 g Protein: 19 g Fat: 1.4 g Sodium: 805 mg Cholesterol: 179 mg

Mango Shrimp

Servings: 4

Cooking Time: 15 Minutes

Ingredients:
- 1lb. shrimp, peeled and deveined but tail intact
- 2tablespoons olive oil
- Mango seasoning

Directions:

1. Turn on your wood pellet grill.
2. Preheat it to 425 degrees F.
3. Coat the shrimp with the oil and season with the mango seasoning.
4. Thread the shrimp into skewers.
5. Grill for 3 minutes per side.
6. Serving Suggestion: Garnish with chopped parsley.

Nutrition Info: Calories: 223.1 Fat: 4.3 g Cholesterol: 129.2 mg Carbohydrates: 29.2 g Fiber: 4.4 g Sugars: 15. 6g Protein: 19.5 g

Cajun Smoked Catfish

Servings: 4

Cooking Time: 2 Hours

Ingredients:
- 4 catfish fillets (5 ounces each)
- ½ cup Cajun seasoning
- 1 tsp ground black pepper
- 1 tbsp smoked paprika
- 1 /4 tsp cayenne pepper
- 1 tsp hot sauce
- 1 tsp granulated garlic
- 1 tsp onion powder
- 1 tsp thyme
- 1 tsp salt or more to taste
- 2 tbsp chopped fresh parsley

Directions:

1. Pour water into the bottom of a square or rectangular dish. Add 4 tbsp salt. Arrange the catfish fillets into the dish. Cover the dish and refrigerate for 3 to 4 hours.

2. Combine the paprika, cayenne, hot sauce, onion, salt, thyme, garlic, pepper and Cajun seasoning in a mixing bowl.

3. Remove the fish from the dish and let it sit for a few minutes, or until it is at room temperature. Pat the fish fillets dry with a paper towel.

4. Rub the seasoning mixture over each fillet generously.

5. Start your grill on smoke, leaving the lid opened for 5 minutes, or until fire starts.

6. Keep lid unopened and preheat to 200°F, using mesquite hardwood pellets.

7. Arrange the fish fillets onto the grill grate and close the grill. Cook for about 2 hours, or until the fish is flaky.

8. Remove the fillets from the grill and let the fillets rest for a few minutes to cool.

9. Serve and garnish with chopped fresh parsley.

Nutrition Info: Calories: 204 Cal Fat: 11.1 g Carbohydrates: 2.7 g Protein: 22.9 g Fiber: 0.6 g

Grilled Lobster Tail

Servings: 4
Cooking Time: 15 Minutes
Ingredients:
- 2 (8 ounces each) lobster tails
- 1/4 tsp old bay seasoning
- ½ tsp oregano
- 1 tsp paprika
- Juice from one lemon
- 1/4 tsp Himalayan salt
- 1/4 tsp freshly ground black pepper
- 1/4 tsp onion powder
- 2 tbsp freshly chopped parsley
- ¼ cup melted butter

Directions:

1. Slice the tail in the middle with a kitchen shear. Pull the shell apart slightly and run your hand through the meat to separate the meat partially

2. Combine the seasonings

3. Drizzle lobster tail with lemon juice and season generously with the seasoning mixture.

4. Preheat your wood pellet smoker to 450°F, using apple wood pellets.

5. Place the lobster tail directly on the grill grate, meat side down. Cook for about 15 minutes.

6. The tails must be pulled off and it must cool down for a few minutes

7. Drizzle melted butter over the tails.

8. Serve and garnish with fresh chopped parsley.

Nutrition Info: Calories: 146 Cal Fat: 11.7 g Carbohydrates: 2.1 g Protein: 9.3 g Fiber: 0.8 g

Hot-smoked Salmon

Servings: 4
Cooking Time: 4 To 6 Hours
Ingredients:
- 1 (2-pound) half salmon fillet
- 1 batch Dill Seafood Rub

Directions:

1. Supply your smoker with wood pellets and follow the manufacturer's specific start-up procedure. Preheat the grill, with the lid closed, to 180°F.

2. Season the salmon all over with the rub. Using your hands, work the rub into the flesh.

3. Place the salmon directly on the grill grate, skin-side down, and smoke until its internal temperature reaches 145°F. Remove the salmon from the grill and serve immediately.

Halibut With Garlic Pesto

Servings: 4

Cooking Time: 10 Minutes

Ingredients:

- 4 halibut fillets
- 1 cup olive oil
- Salt and pepper to taste
- 1/4 cup garlic, chopped
- 1/4 cup pine nuts

Directions:

1. Set the wood pellet grill to smoke.
2. Establish fire for 5 minutes.
3. Set temperature to high.
4. Place a cast iron on a grill.
5. Season fish with salt and pepper.
6. Add fish to the pan.
7. Drizzle with a little oil.
8. Sear for 4 minutes per side.
9. Prepare the garlic pesto by pulsing the remaining ingredients in the food processor until smooth.
10. Serve fish with garlic pesto.
11. Tips: You can also use other white fish fillets for this recipe.

Buttered Crab Legs

Servings: 4

Cooking Time: 10 Minutes

Ingredients:

- 12 tablespoons butter
- 1 tablespoon parsley, chopped
- 1 tablespoon tarragon, chopped
- 1 tablespoon chives, chopped
- 1 tablespoon lemon juice
- 4 lb. king crab legs, split in the center

Directions:

1. Set the wood pellet grill to 375 degrees F.
2. Preheat it for 15 minutes while lid is closed.
3. In a pan over medium heat, simmer the butter, herbs and lemon juice for 2 minutes.
4. Place the crab legs on the grill.
5. Pour half of the sauce on top.
6. Grill for 10 minutes.
7. Serve with the reserved butter sauce.
8. Tips: You can also use shrimp for this recipe.

Spicy Shrimps Skewers

Servings: 4

Cooking Time: 6 Minutes

Ingredients:

- 2 pounds shrimp, peeled, and deveined
- For the Marinade:
- 6 ounces Thai chilies
- 6 cloves of garlic, peeled
- 1 ½ teaspoon sugar
- 2 tablespoons Napa Valley rub
- 1 ½ tablespoon white vinegar
- 3 tablespoons olive oil

Directions:

1. Prepare the marinade and for this, place all of its ingredients in a food processor and then pulse for 1 minute until smooth.
2. Take a large bowl, place shrimps on it, add prepared marinade, toss until well coated, and let marinate for a minimum of 30 minutes in the refrigerator.
3. When ready to cook, switch on the grill, fill the grill hopper with apple-flavored wood pellets, power the grill on by using the control panel, select 'smoke' on the temperature dial, or set the temperature to 450 degrees F and let it preheat for a minimum of 5 minutes.
4. Meanwhile, remove shrimps from the marinade and then thread onto skewers.
5. When the grill has preheated, open the lid, place shrimps' skewers on the grill grate, shut the grill and smoke for 3 minutes per side until firm.
6. When done, transfer shrimps' skewers to a dish and then serve.

Nutrition Info: Calories: 187.2 Cal ;Fat: 2.7 g ;Carbs: 2.7 g ;Protein: 23.2 g ;Fiber: 0.2 g

Seared Tuna Steaks

Servings: 2

Cooking Time: 10 Minutes

Ingredients:

- 2 (1½- to 2-inch-thick) tuna steaks
- 2 tablespoons olive oil
- Salt
- Freshly ground black pepper

Directions:

1. Supply your smoker with wood pellets and follow the manufacturer's specific start-up procedure. Preheat the grill, with the lid closed, to 500°F.

2. Rub the tuna steaks all over with olive oil and season both sides with salt and pepper.

3. Place the tuna steaks directly on the grill grate and grill for 3 to 5 minutes per side, leaving a pink center. Remove the tuna steaks from the grill and serve immediately.

Wood Pellet Smoked Salmon

Servings: 8
Cooking Time: 4 Hours

Ingredients:
- Brine
- 4 cups water
- 1 cup brown sugar
- 1/3 cup kosher salt
- Salmon
- Salmon fillet, skin in
- Maple syrup

Directions:

1. Combine all the brine ingredients until the sugar has fully dissolved.

2. Add the brine to a ziplock bag with the salmon and refrigerate for 12 hours.

3. Remove the salmon from the brine, wash it and rinse with water. Pat dry with paper towel then let sit at room temperature for 2 hours.

4. Startup your wood pellet to smoke and place the salmon on a baking rack sprayed with cooking spray.

5. After cooking for an hour, baste the salmon with maple syrup. Do not let the smoker get above 180°F for accurate results.

6. Smoke for 3-4 hours or until the salmon flakes easily.

Nutrition Info: Calories 101, Total fat 2g, Saturated fat 0g, Total carbs 16g, Net carbs 16g, Protein 4g, Sugar 16g, Fiber 0g, Sodium: 3131mg

OTHER FAVORITE RECIPES

Smoked Cheese Dip

Servings: 8
Cooking Time: 1 Hour And 15 Minutes
Ingredients:
- Ice cubes
- 1 block cheddar cheese
- 8 tablespoons butter
- ½ cup carrots, chopped
- 1 onion, chopped
- 1 cup heavy cream
- 3/4 cup flour
- Hot sauce
- 1 teaspoon Worcestershire sauce

Directions:
1. Preheat your wood pellet grill to 180 degrees F for 15 minutes while the lid is closed.
2. Add ice cubes to a pan.
3. Place a cooling rack on top.
4. Put the cheese block on the rack.
5. Put this on top of the grill.
6. Smoke for 30 minutes.
7. Transfer the cheese to your freezer.
8. In a pan over medium heat, add the butter and let it melt.
9. Cook the onion and carrots for 15 minutes.
10. Stir in the rest of the ingredients.
11. Reduce heat and simmer for 15 minutes.
12. Take the cheese out of the freezer and shred.
13. Put the shredded cheese into the mixture.
14. Stir while cooking until cheese has melted.

Nutrition Info: Calories: 1230 Fats: 77 g Cholesterol: 145 mg Carbohydrates: 104 g Fiber: 8 g Sugar: 7g Protein: 40 g

Smoked Pork Ribs With Fresh Herbs

Servings: 6
Cooking Time: 3 Hours
Ingredients:
- 1/4 cup olive oil
- 1 Tbs garlic minced
- 1 Tbs crushed fennel seeds
- 1 tsp of fresh basil leaves finely chopped
- 1 tsp fresh parsley finely chopped
- 1 tsp fresh rosemary finely chopped
- 1 tsp fresh sage finely chopped
- Salt and ground black pepper to taste
- 3 pounds pork rib roast bone-in

Directions:
1. Combine spices and mix well
2. Coat chop with mixture
3. Start the pellet grill Set temperature to 225 °F and preheat, lid closed, for 10 to 15 minutes. Smoke the ribs for 3 hours. Place the ribs to you preferred container and serve while it is hot

Nutrition Info: Calories: 459.2 Cal Fat: 31.3 g Carbohydrates: 0.6 g Protein: 41 g Fiber: 0.03 g

Chile Cheeseburgers

Servings: 4
Cooking Time: 30 Minutes
Ingredients:
- 1 lb ground chuck (80% lean, 20% fat)
- 4 Monterey Jack cheese slices
- 1/4 cup yellow onion, finely chopped
- 4 hamburger buns
- 2 tbsp hatch chiles, peeled and chopped
- 6 tbsp hatch chile salsa
- 1 tsp kosher salt
- Mayonnaise, to taste
- 1 tsp ground black pepper

Directions:
1. In a bowl, combine beef, diced onion, chopped hatch chiles, salt, and fresh ground pepper. Once evenly mixed, shape into 4 burger patties
2. Preheat pellet grill to 350°FPlace burgers on grill, and cook for about 6 minutes per side or until both sides of each burger are slightly crispy
3. After burger is cooked to desired doneness and both sides have light sear, place cheese slices on each burger. Allow to heat for around 45 seconds or until cheese melts
4. Remove from grill and allow to rest for about 10 minutesSpread a little bit of mayonnaise on both sides of each bun. Place burger patty on bottom side of the bun, then top with hatch chile salsa on top to taste

Smoked Chuck Roast

Servings: 6
Cooking Time: 5 Hours
Ingredients:

- 3 lb. chuck roast
- 3 tablespoons sweet and spicy rub
- 3 cups beef stock, divided
- 1 yellow onion, sliced

Directions:

1. Add the chuck roast to a baking pan.
2. Coat with the sweet, spicy rub.
3. Cover with foil. Refrigerate and marinate overnight.
4. Set the wood pellet grill to smoke.
5. Preheat it to 225 degrees F.
6. Add the chuck roast to the grill.
7. Close the lid.
8. Smoke the chuck roast for 3 hours.
9. Brush with 1 cup beef stock every 1 hour.
10. Add the onion slices to a baking pan.
11. Pour the remaining beef stock.
12. Transfer the chuck roast on top of the onions.
13. Increase the heat to 250 degrees F.
14. Smoke for 3 hours.
15. Cover the chuck roast with the foil.
16. Smoke for another 2 hours and 30 minutes.
17. Let the chuck roast rest for 10 minutes.
18. Serving Suggestion: Serve with mashed potatoes.

Nutrition Info: Calories: 201 Fat: 13 g Cholesterol: 71 mg Carbohydrates: 0 g Fiber: 0 g Sugars: 0 g Protein: 21 g

Cold Hot Smoked Salmon

Servings: 4
Cooking Time: 8 Hours
Ingredients:

- 5 pound of fresh sockeye (red) salmon fillets
- For trout Brine
- 4 cups of filtered water
- 1 cup of soy sauce
- ½ a cup of pickling kosher salt
- ½ a cup of brown sugar
- 2 tablespoon of garlic powder
- 2 tablespoon of onion powder
- 1 teaspoon of cayenne pepper

Directions:

1. Combine all of the ingredients listed under trout brine in two different 1-gallon bags. Store it in your fridge. Cut up the Salmon fillets into 3-4-inch pieces. Place your salmon pieces into your 1-gallon container of trout brine and let it keep in your fridge for 8 hours.
2. Rotate the Salmon and pat them dry using a kitchen towel for 8 hours
3. Configure your pellet smoker for indirect cooking. Remove your salmon pieces of from your fridge Preheat your smoker to a temperature of 180 degrees Fahrenheit
4. Once a cold smoke at 70 degrees Fahrenheit starts smoke your fillets
5. Keep smoking it until the internal temperature reaches 145 degrees Fahrenheit.
6. Remove the Salmon from your smoker and let it rest for 10 minutes

Nutrition Info: Calories: 849 Cal Fat: 45 g Carbohydrates: 51 g Protein: 46 g Fiber: 0 g

Curried Chicken Roast With Tarragon And Custard

Servings: 4
Cooking Time: 1 Hour 45 Minutes
Ingredients:

- 3 Tbsp of olive oil
- 1 Tbsp of salt, kosher
- 1 4pounds chicken
- 1/2 cup of grain mustard, whole
- 3 Tbsp of tarragon, freshly chopped
- 1 tsp of black pepper, freshly ground
- 1 Tbsp of curry powder

Directions:

1. Preheat the grill for direct cooking at 420°F (High). Use hickory wood pellets for a robust taste.
2. Mix the salt, olive oil, mustard, tarragon, pepper, and curry powder in a bowl. Coat the prepared rub all over the chicken with a grill brush. Put the chicken inside a Ziploc bag and refrigerate for an hour.
3. Roast the chicken on the preheated grill for 35 minutes. With a tong, flip the chicken and roast for another 15 minutes, or until the internal temperature of the thigh reads between 168-1690F.

4. Allow cooling for about 10 minutes before slicing and serving.

Nutrition Info: Per Serving: Calories: 330kcal, Protein: 34.1g, Carbs: 48g, Fat: 39g

Smoked Bananas Foster Bread Pudding

Servings: 8 To 10
Cooking Time: 2 Hours 15 Minutes
Ingredients:
- 1loaf (about 4 cups) brioche or challah, cubed to 1 inch cubes
- 3eggs, lightly beaten
- 2cups of milk
- 2/3 cups sugar
- 2large bananas, peeled and smashed
- 1tbsp vanilla extract
- 1tbsp cinnamon
- 1/4 tsp nutmeg
- 1/2 cup pecans
- Rum Sauce Ingredients:
- 1/2 cup spiced rum
- 1/4 cup unsalted butter
- 1cup dark brown sugar
- 1tsp cinnamon
- 5large bananas, peeled and quartered

Directions:
1. Place pecans on a skillet over medium heat and lightly toast for about 5 minutes, until you can smell them.
2. Remove from heat and allow to cool. Once cooled, chop pecans.
3. Lightly butter a 9" x 13" baking dish and evenly layer bread cubes in the dish.
4. In a large bowl, whisk eggs, milk, sugar, mashed bananas, vanilla extract, cinnamon, and nutmeg until combined.
5. Pour egg mixture over the bread in the baking dish evenly. Sprinkle with chopped pecans. Cover with aluminum foil and refrigerate for about 30 minutes.
6. Preheat pellet grill to 180°F. Turn your smoke setting to high, if applicable.
7. Remove foil from dish and place on the smoker for 5 minutes with the lid closed, allowing bread to absorb smoky flavor.

8. Remove dish from the grill and cover with foil again. Increase your pellet grill's temperature to 350°F.
9. Place dish on the grill grate and cook for 50-60 minutes until everything is cooked through and the bread pudding is bubbling.
10. In a saucepan, while pudding cooks heat up butter for rum sauce over medium heat. When the butter begins to melt, add the brown sugar, cinnamon, and bananas. Sauté until bananas begin to soften.
11. Add rum and watch. When the liquid begins to bubble, light a match, and tilt the pan. Slowly and carefully move the match towards the liquid until the sauce lights. When the flames go away, remove skillet from heat.
12. If you're uncomfortable lighting the liquid with a match, just cook it for 3-4 minutes over medium heat after the rum has been added.
13. Keep rum sauce on a simmer or reheat once it's time to serve.
14. Remove bread pudding from the grill and allow it to cool for about 5 minutes.
15. Cut into squares, put each square on a plate and add a piece of banana then drizzle rum sauce over the top. Serve on its own or a la mode and enjoy it!

Nutrition Info: Calories: 274.7 Fat: 7.9 g Cholesterol: 10 mg Carbohydrate: 35.5 g Fiber: 0.9 g Sugar: 24.7 g Protein: 4 g

Seafood On Skewers

Servings: 4
Cooking Time: 40 Minutes
Ingredients:
- 2 Tbsp of peanuts or corn oil
- 16 cubes of swordfish
- 8 sea scallops, big
- Salt and ground pepper, fresh
- 16 cubes of monkfish
- 12 jumbo shrimp
- Sauce Bearnaise

Directions:
1. Set the grill for direct cooking at 200°F. Use oak wood pellets for rich, woody taste.

2. Arrange four pieces of alternating swordfish and monkfish pieces, shrimps, and scallops on a metal skewer. Repeat this for the other three skewers. Rub oil on the skewers.

3. Place the skewers on the preheated grill, and cook for 10 minutes. Flip to the other side and season with salt and pepper. Allow the other side to cook for another 10 minutes. Serve it with béarnaise sauce.

Nutrition Info: Per Serving: Calories: 82kcal, Protein: 20.5g, Fat: 15g, Carb: 16g

Smoked Garlic White Sauce

Servings: 2
Cooking Time: 1 Hour
Ingredients:
- 2 cups hickory wood chips, soaked in water for 30 minutes
- 3 whole garlic heads
- 1/2 cup mayonnaise
- 1/3 cup sour cream
- 1 juiced lemon
- 2 tbsp apple cider vinegar
- Salt to taste

Directions:
1. Cut garlic heads to expose the inside and place in a container, microwave-safe, with 2 tbsp water. Microwave for about 5-6 minutes on medium.
2. Preheat your grill. Place garlic heads on a shallow foil "boat" and place it on the grill.
3. Close the grill and cook for about 20-25 minutes until soft completely. Remove and cool.
4. Transfer into a blender then add the remaining ingredients. Process until smooth.
5. Serve immediately or store in a refrigerator for up to 5 days.

Nutrition Info: Calories 20, Total fat 0g, Saturated fat 0g, Total carbs 8g, Net carbs 8g, Protein 0g, Sugar 0g, Fiber 0g, Sodium: 45mg

Garlic Aioli And Smoked Salmon Sliders

Servings: 12
Cooking Time: 1 Hour And 30 Minutes
Ingredients:
- For Brine:

- Water as needed
- ½ a cup of salt
- 1 tablespoon of dried tarragon
- 1 and a ½ pound of salmon fillets
- For Aioli:
- 1 cup of mayonnaise
- 3 tablespoon of fresh lemon juice
- 3 minced garlic cloves
- 1 and a ½ teaspoon of ground black pepper
- ½ a teaspoon of lemon zest
- Salt as needed
- ½ a cup of apple wood chips
- 12 slide burger buns

Directions:
1. Take a large sized baking dish and add ½ a cup of salt alongside about half water
2. Add tarragon, salmon in the brine mix and keep adding more water
3. Cover up the dish and freeze for 2-12 hours. Take a small bowl and add lemon juice, mayonnaise, pepper, garlic, 1 pinch of salt and lemon zest.
4. Mix and chill for 30 minutes
5. Remove your Salmon from the brine and place it on a wire rack and let it sit for about 30 minutes.
6. Smoke them over low heat for 1 and a ½ to 2 hours. Assemble sliders by dividing the salmon among 12 individual buns.
7. Top each of the pieces with a spoonful of aioli and place another bun on top

Nutrition Info: Calories: 320 Cal Fat: 22 g Carbohydrates: 13 g   Protein: 22 g Fiber: 0 g

Smoked Chicken With Perfect Poultry Rub

Servings: 2
Cooking Time: 3 Hours 15 Minutes
Ingredients:
- 2 Tbsp of onion, powder
- 1/4 cup of black pepper, freshly ground
- 2 Tbsp of dry mustard
- 3/4 cup of paprika
- 4pound chicken
- 3 lemon
- 2 tsp of cayenne
- 1/4 cup of sugar
- 1/4 cup of celery salt

Directions:

1. In a bowl, mix the onion powder, paprika, black pepper, dry mustard, cayenne, sugar, celery, salt, and 2 lemons.
2. Add your chicken to the rub and slice some parts so that the ingredients will find their way in.
3. Preheat the grill for 15 minutes at 225°F. Use apple wood pellets for a distinctive, strong woody taste.
4. Place the coated chicken on the preheated grill and smoke for 3 hours or until internal temperature reads 160°F.
5. Allow chicken to cool, then serve.

Nutrition Info: Per Serving: Calories: 255kcal, Protein: 35g, Carbs: 42g, Fat: 35g.

Pizza Bianca

Servings: 2
Cooking Time: 3 Hours
Ingredients:

- 3cups all-purpose or bread flour, plus more as needed
- 2teaspoons instant yeast
- 2teaspoons kosher or coarse sea salt, plus more for sprinkling
- 2tablespoons good-quality olive oil, plus more for drizzling
- 1tablespoon or more chopped fresh rosemary

Directions:

1. Whisk the flour, yeast, and salt together in a large bowl. Add the oil and 1 cup water and mix with a heavy spoon. Continue to add water, 1 tablespoon at a time, until the dough forms a ball and is slightly sticky to the touch. In the unlikely event that the mixture gets too sticky, add flour 1 tablespoon at a time until you have the right consistency.
2. Lightly flour a work surface and turn out the dough onto it. Knead by hand for a minute until smooth, then form into a round ball. Put the dough in a bowl and cover with plastic wrap; let rise in a warm spot until it doubles in size, 1 to 2 hours. You can cut this rising time short if you're in a hurry, or you can let the dough rise more slowly, in the refrigerator, for up to 8 hours. You can freeze the dough at this point for up to a month: Wrap it tightly in plastic wrap or put in a zipper bag. Thaw in the refrigerator; bring to room temperature before shaping.
3. To shape, divide the dough into 2 or more pieces; roll each piece into a round ball. Put each ball on a lightly floured work surface, sprinkle lightly with flour, and cover with plastic wrap or a towel. Let rest until slightly puffed, 25 to 30 minutes.
4. Start the coals or heat a gas grill for medium direct cooking. Make sure the grates are clean.
5. Roll or lightly press each ball into a flat, round disk, lightly flouring the work surface and the dough as necessary to keep it from sticking (use only as much flour as you need). To stretch the dough, push down at the center and outward to the edge, turning the round as you do. Continue pushing down and out and turning the dough until the round is the size you want; if you're making 2 pizzas, aim for rounds 10 to 12 inches in diameter. Sprinkle the tops evenly with the rosemary and a pinch or so coarse salt, then drizzle with olive oil.
6. Put the crusts on the grill directly over the fire. Close the lid and cook until the bottoms firm up and brown and the tops are cooked through, 5 to 10 minutes, depending on how hot the fire is; the top side of the dough will bubble up from the heat underneath but likely won't take on much color. Transfer to a cutting board and use a pizza cutter to slice into wedges or small pieces and serve.

Nutrition Info: Calories: 460 Fats: 17 g Cholesterol: 20 mg Carbohydrates: 56 g Fiber: 3 g Sugars: 7 g Proteins: 18 g

Barbecue Sandwich

Servings: 6
Cooking Time: 30 Minutes
Ingredients:

- 3 lb. steak
- ½ cup barbecue sauce
- 6 ciabatta rolls
- 6 slices cheddar cheese

Directions:

1. Preheat your wood pellet grill to 450 degrees F. for 15 minutes while the lid is closed.
2. Grill the steak for 30 minutes.
3. Let rest on a cutting board.
4. Slice thinly.

5. Coat with the barbecue sauce.
6. Stuff in ciabatta rolls with cheese.
7. Tips: You can also smoke the beef before grilling.

Reverse-seared Tilapia

Servings: 4
Cooking Time: 20 Minutes
Ingredients:
- tilapia fillets
- 2 Tbsp melted butter (unsalted)
- 1/2 cup of all-purpose flour
- Salt and pepper to taste

Directions:
1. Preheat the wood pellet smoker-grill for direct cooking at 350 F using any pellet
2. Rinse the fillets and pat dry with a paper towel. Season with salt and pepper, coat with the flour.
3. Transfer Tilapia fillets to cooking grate and grill for 20 minutes or until internal temperature measure 150 F. Then set fillets aside and increase the temperature of the grill to 450 F
4. Sear the tilapia for 4 minutes per side or until it flakes. Brush melted butter on the tilapia.
5. Serve.
Nutrition Info: Per Serving: Calories: 295kcal, Carbs: 11.2g, Fat: 16g, Protein: 24.6g

Cornish Game Hens

Servings: 6
Cooking Time: 1 Hour
Ingredients:
- 4 Cornish game hens, giblets removed
- 4 teaspoons chicken rub
- 4 sprigs of rosemary
- 4 tablespoons butter, unsalted, melted

Directions:
1. Switch on the grill, fill the grill hopper with mesquite flavored wood pellets, power the grill on by using the control panel, select 'smoke' on the temperature dial, or set the temperature to 375 degrees F and let it preheat for a minimum of 15 minutes.
2. Meanwhile, rinse the hens, pat dry with paper towels, tie the wings by using a butcher's strong, then rub evenly with melted butter, sprinkle with chicken rub and stuff cavity of each hen with a rosemary sprig.
3. When the grill has preheated, open the lid, place hens on the grill grate, shut the grill, and smoke for 1 hour until thoroughly cooked and internal temperature reaches 165 degrees F.
4. When done, transfer hens to a dish, let rest for 5 minutes and then serve.
Nutrition Info: Calories: 173 Cal ;Fat: 7.4 g ;Carbs: 1 g ;Protein: 24.1 g ;Fiber: 0.2 g

Black Bean Dipping Sauce

Servings: 4
Cooking Time: 10 Minutes
Ingredients:
- 2 tablespoons black bean paste
- 2 tablespoons peanut butter
- 1 tablespoon maple syrup
- 2 tablespoons olive oil

Directions:
1. In a blender place all ingredients and blend until smooth
2. Pour sauce in a bowl and serve

Roasted Ham

Servings: 12
Cooking Time: 6 Hours
Ingredients:
- 2 quarts water
- 1/2 cup quick home meat cure
- 1/2 cup kosher salt
- 3/4 cup brown sugar
- 1 tablespoon pork rub
- 1 teaspoon whole cloves
- 10 lb. fresh ham
- 1 teaspoon whole cloves
- 1/4 cup pure maple syrup
- 2 cup apple juice

Directions:
1. In a large container, pour in the water and add the meat cure, salt, sugar, pork rub and whole cloves.
2. Mix well.
3. Soak the ham in the brine.

4. Cover and refrigerate for 1 day.
5. Rinse ham with water and dry with paper towels.
6. Score the ham with crosshatch pattern.
7. Insert remaining cloves into the ham.
8. Season ham with the pork rub.
9. Add ham to a roasting pan.
10. Smoke the ham in the wood pellet grill for 2 hours at 180 degrees F.
11. Make the glaze by mixing the maple syrup and apple juice.
12. Brush the ham with this mixture.
13. Increase heat to 300 degrees F.
14. Roast for 4 hours.
15. Tips: You can also inject the brine into the ham.

Polish Kielbasa

Servings: 8
Cooking Time: 1 To 2 Hours
Ingredients:
- 4 pounds ground pork
- ½ cup water
- 2 garlic cloves, minced
- 4 teaspoons salt
- 1 teaspoon freshly ground black pepper
- 1 teaspoon dried marjoram
- ½ teaspoon ground allspice
- 14 feet natural hog casings, medium size

Directions:
1. In a large bowl, combine the pork, water, garlic, salt, pepper, marjoram, and allspice.
2. Stuff the casings according to the instructions on your sausage stuffing device, or use a funnel (see Tip).
3. Twist the casings according to your desired length and prick each with a pin in several places so the kielbasa won't burst.
4. Transfer the kielbasa to a plate, cover with plastic wrap, and refrigerate for at least 8 hours or overnight.
5. Remove from the refrigerator and allow the links to come to room temperature.
6. Supply your smoker with wood pellets and follow the manufacturer's specific start-up procedure. Preheat, with the lid closed, to 225°F.
7. Place the kielbasa directly on the grill grate, close the lid, and smoke for 1 hour 30 minutes to 2 hours, or until a meat thermometer inserted in each link reads 155°F. (The internal temperature will rise about 5°F when resting, for a finished temp of 160°F.)
8. Serve with buns and condiments of your choosing, or cut up the kielbasa and serve with smoked cabbage

Super-addicting Mushrooms

Servings: 4
Cooking Time: 45 Minutes
Ingredients:
- 4 C. fresh whole baby Portobello mushrooms, cleaned
- 1 tbsp. canola oil
- 1 tsp. granulated garlic
- 1 tsp. onion powder
- Salt and freshly ground black pepper, to taste

Directions:
1. Set the temperature of Grill to 180 degrees F and preheat with closed lid for 15 minutes, using charcoal.
2. In a bowl, add all ingredients and mix well.
3. Place the mushrooms onto the grill and cook for about 30 minutes.
4. Remove the mushrooms from grill.
5. Now, preheat the Grill to 400 degrees F and preheat with closed lid for 15 minutes.
6. Place the mushrooms onto the grill and cook for about 15 minutes.
7. Remove the mushrooms from grill and serve warm.

Nutrition Info: Calories per serving: 50; Carbohydrates: 3.3g; Protein: 2.4g; Fat: 3.7g; Sugar: 1.6g; Sodium: 43mg; Fiber: 0.8g

Pork Fennel Burger

Servings: 4
Cooking Time: 30 Minutes
Ingredients:
- 1 fennel bulb, trimmed and cut into large chunks
- 3 to 4 garlic cloves
- 2 ½ pounds boneless pork shoulder, with some of the fat, cut into 1-inch cubes
- 1 tablespoon fennel seeds

- 1 teaspoon caraway seeds (optional)
- 1 teaspoon salt
- ½ teaspoon pepper, or more to taste
- Peeled orange slices to garnish (optional)
- Chopped olives to garnish (optional)
- Chopped parsley to garnish (optional)
- Chopped roasted red pepper to garnish (optional)
- Fennel slices, to garnish (optional)

Directions:
1. Put fennel and garlic into a food processor and pulse until just chopped; remove to a large bowl. Put pork fat in processor and grind until just chopped; add to bowl. Working in batches, process meat with fennel seeds, caraway, if using and salt and pepper, until meat is just chopped (be careful not to over-process). Add to bowl and mix well. Shape mixture into 8 patties.
2. Supply your smoker with wood pellets and follow the manufacturer's specific start-up procedure. Preheat, with the lid closed, to 425°FArrange the burgers directly on one side of the grill, close the lid, and smoke for 10 minutes. Flip and smoke with the lid closed for 10 to 15 minutes more, or until a meat thermometer inserted in the burgers reads 160°F. Add another Gruyère slice to the burgers during the last 5 minutes of smoking to melt.
3. Garnish with peeled orange slices, chopped olives, chopped parsley, chopped roasted red pepper and fennel slices, to taste.

Spiced Nuts

Servings: 32
Cooking Time: 20 Minutes
Ingredients:
- 1teaspoon dried rosemary
- 1/8 teaspoon cayenne pepper
- 1/8 teaspoon ground black pepper
- ½ teaspoon salt or to taste
- ½ teaspoon ground cuminutes
- 1tablespoon olive oil
- 2tablespoon maple syrup
- 2/3 cup raw and unsalted cashew nuts
- 2/3 cup raw and unsalted pecans
- 2/3 cup raw and unsalted walnuts

Directions:
1. Start your grill on smoke mode, leaving the lid open for 5 minutes, until the fire starts.
2. Close the grill lid and preheat the grill to 350°F.
3. In a large bowl, combine all the ingredients except the dried rosemary. Mix thoroughly until the ingredients are evenly mixed, and all nuts are coated with spices.
4. Spread the spiced nuts on a baking sheet.
5. Place the baking sheet on the grill and roast the nuts for 20 to 25 minutes.
6. Remove the nuts from heat.
7. Sprinkle the dried rosemary on the nuts and stir to mix.
8. Leave the nuts to cool for a few minutes.
9. Serve and enjoy.

Nutrition Info: Calories: 64 Total Fat: 5.8 g Saturated Fat: 0.4 g Cholesterol: 0 mg Sodium: 35 mg Total Carbohydrate 2.2 g Dietary Fiber 0.6 g Total Sugars: 0.8 g Protein: 1.3 g

Grilled Bacon Dog

Servings: 4 To 6
Cooking Time: 25 Minutes
Ingredients:
- 16 Hot Dogs
- 16 Slices Bacon, sliced
- 2 Onion, sliced
- 16 hot dog buns
- As Needed The Ultimate BBQ Sauce
- As Needed Cheese

Directions:
1. When ready to cook, set the to 375°F and preheat, lid closed for 15 minutes.
2. Wrap bacon strips around the hot dogs, and grill directly on the grill grate for 10 minutes each side. Grill onions at the same time as the hot dogs, and cook for 10 -15 minutes.
3. Open hot dog buns and spread BBQ sauce, the grilled hot dogs, cheese sauce and grilled onions. Top with vegetables. Serve, enjoy!

Roasted Almonds

Servings: 6

Cooking Time: 1 Hour And 30 Minutes

Ingredients:

- 1 egg white
- Salt to taste
- 1 tablespoon ground cinnamon
- 1 cup granulated sugar
- 1 lb. almonds

Directions:

1. Beat the egg white in a bowl until frothy.
2. Stir in salt, cinnamon and sugar.
3. Coat the almonds with this mixture.
4. Spread almonds on a baking pan.
5. Set your wood pellet grill to 225 degrees F.
6. Preheat for 15 minutes while the lid is closed.
7. Roast the almonds for 90 minutes, stirring every 10 minutes.
8. Tips: Store in an airtight container with lid for up to 1 week.

Steak Sauce

Servings: ½ Cup
Cooking Time: 25 Minutes

Ingredients:

- Tbsp Malt vinegar
- 1/2 tsp Salt
- 1/2 tsp black pepper
- Tbsp Tomato sauce
- 2 Tbsp brown sugar
- 1 tsp hot pepper sauce
- 2 Tbsp Worcestershire sauce
- 2 Tbsp Raspberry jam.

Directions:

1. Preheat your grill for indirect cooking at 150°F
2. Place a saucepan over grates, add all your ingredients, and allow to boil.
3. Reduce the temperature to Smoke and allow the sauce to simmer for 10 minutes or until sauce is thick.

Nutrition Info: Per Serving: Calories: 62.1kcal, Carbs: 15.9g Fat: 0.3g, Protein:0.1g

Native Southern Cornbread

Servings: 8
Cooking Time: 20 Minutes

Ingredients:

- 2 tbsp. butter
- 1½ C. all-purpose flour
- 1½ C. yellow cornmeal
- 2 tbsp. sugar
- 3 tsp. baking powder
- ¾ tsp. baking soda
- ¾ tsp. salt
- 1 C. whole milk
- 1 C. buttermilk
- 3 large eggs
- 3 tbsp. butter, melted

Directions:

1. Set the temperature of Grill to 400 degrees F and preheat with closed lid for 15 minutes.
2. In a 13x9-inch baking dish, place 2 tbsp. of butter.
3. Place the baking dish onto grill to melt butter and heat up the pan.
4. In a large bowl, mix together flour, cornmeal, sugar, baking powder, baking soda and salt.
5. In another bowl, add milk, buttermilk, eggs and melted butter and beat until well combined.
6. Add the egg mixture into flour mixture and mix until just moistened.
7. Carefully, remove the heated baking dish from grill.
8. Place the bread mixture into heated baking dish evenly.
9. Place the pan onto the grill and cook for about 20 minutes or until a toothpick inserted in the center comes out clean.
10. Remove from grill and place the pan onto a wire rack to cool for about 10 minutes.
11. Carefully, invert the bread onto the wire rack to cool completely before slicing.
12. Cut the bread into desired-sized slices and sere.

Nutrition Info: Calories per serving: 302; Carbohydrates: 42.4g; Protein: 8.7g; Fat: 10.4g; Sugar: 6.4g; Sodium: 467mg; Fiber: 2.3g

Buttered Green Peas

Servings: 1-2
Cooking Time: 30 Minutes

Ingredients:

- 1/2 cup butter, melted

- Kosher salt
- 24 oz green beans, trimmed
- 1/4 cup veggie rub

Directions:

1. Preheat the wood pellet smoker-grill to 345°F using pellets of your choice
2. Pour the beans into a baking pan lined with parchment sheets and rub melted butter over the beans. Season with salt. Place the baking pan on the cooking grid.
3. Arrange the beans on the pan with a tong and pour the veggie rub over it.
4. Braise the beans until tender and lightly browned. Flip after 20 minutes.
5. Serve.

Nutrition Info: Per Serving: Calories: 93kcal, Carbs: 9.5g, Fat: 3.8g, Protein: 3.8g

Twice-baked Spaghetti Squash

Servings: 2
Cooking Time: 1 Hour 15 Minutes
Ingredients:

- 1 medium spaghetti squash
- 1/2 cup of parmesan cheese (grated and divided)
- 1/2 cup of mozzarella cheese (shredded and divided)
- 1 tsp Salt
- Tbsp Extra-virgin olive oil
- 1/2 tsp Pepper

Directions:

1. Set the wood pellet smoker-grill to indirect cooking at 375 F
2. Using a knife, cut the squash into half lengthwise and remove the seed and pulp. Rub the inside of the squash with olive oil, salt, and pepper. Place on the hot grill with the open part facing up and bake for 45 minutes or until the squash can be easily pierced with a fork. Remove and allow to cool.
3. Place on a cutting board. Using a fork, scrape across the surface in a lengthwise direction to remove the flesh-in strand (to look like spaghetti). Transfer to a bowl, add parmesan and mozzarella cheese, then stir well. Stuff back into the shell, sprinkle cheese on the toppings.

4. Increase the pellet smoker-grill to 425 F, place the stuffed squash on the hot grill and bake for 15 minutes or until cheese starts to brown.
5. Remove and allow to cool, serve.

Nutrition Info: Per Serving: Calories: 294kcal, Carbs: 10.1g, Fat:12g, Protein: 16g

Avocado Smoothie

Servings: 2
Cooking Time: 5 Minutes
Ingredients:

- 1 cup Coconut Milk, preferably full-fat
- 1 cup Ice
- 3 cups Baby Spinach
- 1 Banana, frozen and quartered
- 1/2 cup pineapple chunks, frozen
- 1/2 of 1 Avocado, smooth

Directions:

1. First, place ice, pineapple chunks, pineapple chunks, banana, avocado, baby spinach in the blender pitcher.
2. Now, press the 'extract' button.
3. Finally, transfer to a serving glass.

Nutrition Info: Fat: 25.1 g Calories: 323 Total Carbs: 29.2 g Fiber: 11.4 g Sugar: 8.3 g Protein: 5.1 g Cholesterol: 0

Pan-seared Pork Tenderloin With Apple Mashed Potatoes

Servings: 6
Cooking Time: 20 Minutes
Ingredients:

- 2 pork tenderloin
- medium potatoes (peeled and sliced)
- 3 Tbsp unsalted butter
- 1/2 cup of heavy cream
- 2 Tbsp Olive oil
- 1-1/2 Tbsp Pepper
- 1-1/2 Tbsp Salt.
- 2 apple (cored and sliced)

Directions:

1. Preheat the wood pellet smoker-grill for direct cooking at 300 F using any pellet.

2. Season the pork with salt and pepper, then roast meat for 20 minutes.

3. Increase the temperature of the grill to High, then place an iron skillet on the grates, and add 1 Tbsp butter and oil. Cook until the butter becomes brown, make sure it does not burn.

4. Place the tenderloin and cook for 4 minutes per side or until it is brown, transfer to a baking sheet and bake for 10 minutes.

5. Rearrange the grill for indirect cooking at 300 F

6. Place a pot over the cooking grid and fill it with water. Add potatoes and allow to boil, reduce the heat and simmer for 8 minutes or until soft. Drain the water

7. Pour the potatoes into a food processor, add cream and butter. Puree the mixture, add the apples and puree until they are finely chopped. Season with salt and pepper and serve with the pork.

Nutrition Info: Per Serving: Calories: 477kcal, Carbs: 26.9g, Fat: 24.5g, Protein: 46.5g

Smoked Teriyaki Tuna

Servings: 4
Cooking Time: 2 Hours
Ingredients:
- Tuna steaks, 1 oz.
- 2 c. marinade, teriyaki
- Alder wood chips soaked in water

Directions:
1. Slice tuna into thick slices of 2 inch. Place your tuna slices and marinade then set in your fridge for about 3 hours

2. After 3 hours, remove the tuna from the marinade and pat dry. Let the tuna air dry in your fridge for 2-4 hours. Preheat your smoker to 180 degrees Fahrenheit

3. Place the Tuna on a Teflon-coated fiberglass and place them directly on your grill grates. Smoke the Tuna for about an hour until the internal temperature reaches 145 degrees Fahrenheit.

4. Remove the tuna from your grill and let them rest for 10 minutes. Serve!

Nutrition Info: Calories: 249 Cal Fat: 3 g Carbohydrates: 33 g   Protein: 21 g Fiber: 0 g

Sweet Sensation Pork Meat

Servings: 3
Cooking Time: 3 Hours
Ingredients:
- 2 tsp of nutmeg, ground
- 1/4 cup of allspice
- 2 tsp of thyme, dried
- 1/4 cup of brown sugar
- 2 pounds of pork
- 2 tsp of cinnamon, ground
- 2 Tbsp of salt, kosher or sea

Directions:
1. Preheat the grill for 15 minutes at 225°F. Use hickory wood pellets

2. Combine all the ingredients (except pork) in a bowl. Mix thoroughly.

3. Slice the sides of the pork meat in 4-5 places. Put some of the ingredients into the slices and rub the rest over the pork.

4. Place the pork on the preheated grill and smoke for 3 hours or until internal temperature reads 145°F.

5. Allow it to rest before serving.

Nutrition Info: Per Serving: Calories: 300kcal, Protein: 36g, Carbs: 45g, Fat: 31g

Hickory Smoked Green Beans

Servings: 10
Cooking Time: 3 Hours
Ingredients:
- 6 cups fresh green beans, halved and ends cut off
- 2 cups chicken broth
- 1 tbsp pepper, ground
- 1/4 tbsp salt
- 2 tbsp apple cider vinegar
- 1/4 cup diced onion
- 6-8 bite-size bacon slices
- Optional: sliced almonds

Directions:
1. Add green beans to a colander then rinse thoroughly. Set aside.

2. Place chicken broth, pepper, salt, and apple cider in a pan, large. Add green beans.

3. Blanch over medium heat for about 3-4 minutes then remove from heat.

4. Transfer the mixture into an aluminum pan, disposable. Make sure all mixture goes into the pan, so do not drain them.

5. Place bacon slices over the beans and place the pan into the wood pellet smoker,

6. Smoke for about 3 hours uncovered.

7. Remove from the smoker and top with almonds slices.

8. Serve immediately.

Nutrition Info: Calories: 57 Total Fat: 3 g Saturated Fat: 1 g Total Carbs: 6 g Net Carbs: 4 g Protein: 4 g Sugars: 2 g Fiber: 2 g Sodium: 484 mg

Banana Walnut Bread

Servings: 1
Cooking Time: 1 Hour 15 Minutes
Ingredients:
- 2-1/2 cup of all-purpose flour
- 1 cup of sugar
- 2 eggs
- 1 cup ripe banana, mashed
- 1/4 cup whole milk
- 1/4 cup walnut, finely chopped
- 1 tsp salt
- 3 Tbsp of Vegetable oil
- 3 tsp baking powder

Directions:
1. Set the wood pellet smoker-grill for indirect cooking at 350 F.

2. Combine all the ingredients in a large bowl. Using a mixer (electric or manual), mix the ingredients. Grease and flour the loaf pan. Pour the mixture into the loaf pan.

3. Transfer loaf pan to the grill and cover with steel construction. Bake for 60-75 minutes. Remove and allow to cool.

Nutrition Info: Per Serving: Calories: 548kcal, Carbs: 69g, Fat: 36g, Protein: 14g

Empanadas

Servings: 4
Cooking Time: 20 Minutes
Ingredients:
- 3/4 cup + 1 tbsp all-purpose flour
- ½ tsp baking powder
- 1tbsp sugar
- ¼ tsp salt or to taste
- 2tbsp cold water
- 1/3 cups butter
- 1small egg (beaten)
- Filling:
- ½ small onion (chopped)
- 57 g ground beef (1/8 pound)
- 2tbsp marinara sauce
- 1small carrot peeled and diced)
- 1/8 small potato (peeled and diced) 35 grams
- 2tbsp water
- 1garlic clove (minced)
- 1tbsp olive oil
- 1tbsp raisin
- 2tbsp green peas
- ½ tsp salt or taste
- 1/2 tsp ground black pepper or to taste
- 1hard-boiled egg (sliced)

Directions:
1. Start your grill on smoke mode and leave the lid open for 5 minutes, or until fire starts.

2. Close the grill and preheat grill to 400°F with the lid closed for 15 minutes, using hickory hardwood pellets.

3. For the fillet, place a cast iron skillet on the grill and add the oil.

4. Once the oil is hot, add the onion and garlic and sauté until the onion is tender and translucent.

5. Add the ground beef and sauté until it is tender, stirring often.

6. Stir in the marinara, salt, water, and pepper.

7. Bring to a boil and reduce the heat. Cook for 30 seconds.

8. Stir in the carrot, raisin, and potatoes and cook for 3 minutes.

9. Stir in the green peas and sliced egg. Cook for additional 2 minutes, stirring often.

10. Spray a baking dish with a non-stick spray.

11. For the dough, combine the flour, baking powder salt and sugar in a large mixing bowl. Mix until well combined.

12. Add butter and mix until it is well incorporated.

13. Add egg and mix until you form the dough.

14. Put the dough on a floured surface and knead the dough for a few minutes. Add more flour if the dough is not thick enough.

15. Roll the dough flat with a rolling pin. The flat dough should be ¼ inch thick.

16. Cut the flat dough into circles.

17. Add equal amounts of the beef mixture to the middle of each flat circular dough slice. Fold the dough slice and close the edges by pressing with your fingers or a fork.

18. Arrange the empanadas into the baking sheet in a single layer.

19. Place the baking sheet on the grill and bake for 10 minutes.

20. Remove the baking sheet from the grill and flip the empanadas.

21. Bake for another 10 minutes on the grill or until empanadas are golden brown.

Nutrition Info: Calories: 353 Total Fat: 22.3 g Saturated Fat: 11.3 g Cholesterol: 129 mg Sodium: 481 mg Total Carbohydrate 28.9 g Dietary Fiber 1.9 g Total Sugars: 6.6 g Protein: 10.4 g

Cumin Salt

Servings: 1/4 Cup
Cooking Time: 5 Minutes
Ingredients:
- 1 teaspoon cumin seeds
- ¼ cup medium-coarse or flaky sea salt
- Pinch red pepper flakes (optional)
- Pinch cayenne or hot paprika (optional)

Directions:
1. Toast cumin seeds in a dry skillet over medium-high heat until fragrant and lightly colored, about 1 minute.
2. Grind very coarsely in a mortar or spice mill.
3. Combine in a bowl with salt and stir together.
4. Add red pepper flakes or cayenne, if using.

Marinated Chicken Kabobs

Servings: 6
Cooking Time: 12 Minutes
Ingredients:
- Marinade

- 1/2 cup olive oi
- 2 tbsp white vinegar
- 1 tbsp lemon juice
- 1-1/2 tbsp salt
- 1/2 tbsp ground pepper
- 2 tbsp fresh chives, chopped
- 1-1/2 tbsp thyme, chopped
- 2 tbsp Italian parsley, chopped
- 1 tbsp minced garlic
- Kabobs
- 1-1/2 lb chicken breast
- 12 crimini mushrooms
- 1 each orange, red and yellow bell pepper
- Serve with
- Naan bread

Directions:
1. Mix all the marinade ingredients then toss the chicken and mushrooms until well coated.
2. Place in the fridge to marinate for 30 minutes.
3. Meanwhile, soak the skewers in water. And preheat your to 450F.
4. Assemble the kabobs and grill for 6 minutes on each side. Set aside.
5. Heat up the naan bread on the grill for 2 minutes .serve and enjoy.

Nutrition Info: Calories 165, Total fat 5g, Saturated fat 2g, Total carbs 1g, Net carbs 1g Protein 0g, Sugars 0g, Fiber 0g, Sodium 582mg

Potluck Favorite Baked Beans

Servings: 10
Cooking Time: 3 Hours 5 Minutes
Ingredients:
- 1 tbsp. butter
- ½ of red bell pepper, seeded and chopped
- ½ of medium onion, chopped
- 2 jalapeño peppers, chopped
- 2 (28-oz.) cans baked beans, rinsed and drained
- 8 oz. pineapple chunks, drained
- 1 C. BBQ sauce
- 1 C. brown sugar
- 1 tbsp. ground mustard

Directions:
1. Set the temperature of Grill to 220-250 degrees F and preheat with closed lid for 15 minutes.

2.   In a non-stick skillet, melt butter over medium heat and sauté the bell peppers, onion and jalapeño peppers for about 4-5 minutes.

3.   Remove from heat and transfer the pepper mixture into a bowl.

4.   Add remaining ingredients and stir to combine.

5.   Transfer the mixture into a Dutch oven.

6.   Place the Dutch oven onto the grill and cook for about 2½-3 hours.

7.   Remove from grill and serve hot.

Nutrition Info: Calories per serving: 364; Carbohydrates: 61.4g; Protein: 9.4g; Fat: 9.8g; Sugar: 23.5g; Sodium: 1036mg; Fiber: 9.7g

Red Wine Beef Stew

Servings: 8
Cooking Time: 3 Hours 30 Minutes
Ingredients:
- 1-1/2 tsp kosher salt
- 4lb chuck roast, cut into 2-inch pieces
- 1 Tsp ground black pepper
- 1/4 cup tomato paste
- 1 Tsp olive oil
- 2 cups dry red wine
- 2 bay leaves
- 4 spring's fresh thyme
- 2 lb carrots, peeled and chopped
- 1lb red potatoes, cut into half
- 4 cups chicken broth
- 3 Tsp all-purpose flour

Directions:
1.   Preheat wood pellet smoker-grill to 325^{0}F, with the lid closed for about 15 minutes

2.   Place meat in a bowl and sprinkle in salt, pepper, and flour. Toss together until meat is adequately seasoned.

3.   Heat oil in a cast-iron Dutch oven and cook the meat at Medium for about 8 minutes, until brown.

4.   Remove meat and place on a plate. Add wine, broth, tomato paste, thyme, bay leaves, and 1/4 of carrots into the Dutch oven and bring to a boil. Transfer meat to Dutch oven and place on the grill grate for direct cooking. Cook meat for about 2 hours.

5.   Remove cooked vegetables from Dutch oven and add remaining carrots and potatoes. Cook until meat is fork-tender, about 1 hour.

6.   Serve.

Nutrition Info: Per Serving: Calories: 402kcal, Carbs: 17.3g, Fat: 15.4g, Protein: 35.5g

Seafaring Seafood Rub With Smoked Swordfish

Servings: 6-8
Cooking Time: 2 Hours 15 Minutes
Ingredients:
- 4 tsp of garlic, ground
- 2 tsp of paprika
- 1 tsp of nutmeg, ground
- 1/2 tsp of allspice, ground
- 4 tsp of ginger, ground
- 1 tsp of cayenne
- 2 Tbsp of celery seed
- 1/4 cup of sea salt
- 4 tsp of black pepper, freshly ground
- 2 pounds of swordfish
- 2 tsp of brown sugar

Directions:
1.   Preheat the grill for 15 minutes at 225°F. Use oak wood pellets for a distinctive, strong woody taste.

2.   Combine all the ingredients (except swordfish) in a bowl. Mix thoroughly.

3.   Add the swordfish to the bowl and gently coat it with the mixture. Do not allow the swordfish to break.

4.   Place the coated swordfish directly on the preheated grate and smoke for 2 hours or until fish turns opaque and flakes.

5.   Serve immediately.

Nutrition Info: Per Serving: Calories: 173kcal, Carbs: 27g, Protein: 21.9g, Fat:19g.

Smoked Tuna

Servings: 6
Cooking Time: 3 Hours
Ingredients:
- 2 cups water
- 1 cup brown sugar

- 1 cup salt
- 1 tablespoon lemon zest
- 6 tuna fillets

Directions:

1. Mix water, brown sugar, salt and lemon zest in a bowl.
2. Coat the tuna fillets with the mixture.
3. Refrigerate for 6 hours.
4. Rinse the tuna and pat dry with paper towels.
5. Preheat the wood pellet grill to 180 degrees F for 15 minutes while the lid is closed.
6. Smoke the tuna for 3 hours.
7. Tips: You can also soak tuna in the brine for 24 hours.

Wood Pellet Spicy Brisket

Servings: 10
Cooking Time: 9 Hours
Ingredients:

- 2 tbsp garlic powder
- 2 tbsp onion powder
- 2 tbsp paprika
- 2 tbsp chili powder
- 1/3 cup salt
- 1/3 cup black pepper
- 12 lb whole packer brisket, trimmed
- 1-1/2 cup beef broth

Directions:

1. Set your wood pellet temperature to 225°F. Let preheat for 15 minutes with the lid closed.
2. Meanwhile, mix garlic, onion, paprika, chili, salt, and pepper in a mixing bowl.
3. the brisket generously on all sides.
4. Place the meat on the grill with the fat side down and let it cool until the internal temperature reaches 160°F.
5. Remove the meat from the grill and double wrap it with foil. Return it to the grill and cook until the internal temperature reaches 204°F.
6. Remove from grill, unwrap the brisket and let rest for 15 minutes.
7. Slice and serve.

Nutrition Info: Calories: 270 Total Fat: 20 g Saturated Fat: 8 g Total Carbs: 3 g Net Carbs: 3 g Protein: 20 g Sugar: 1 g Fiber: 0 g Sodium: 1220mg

Banana Nut Oatmeal

Servings: 2
Cooking Time: 5 Minutes
Ingredients:

- 1/2 tbsp. Maple Syrup
- 1/4 cup Hemp Seeds
- 1/2 cup Steel Cut Oats
- Dash of Sea Salt
- 1 tsp. Vanilla Extract
- 1/2 cup Water
- 1/2 tsp. Cinnamon
- 1 tsp. Nutmeg
- 1/3 cup Milk
- 1 Banana, medium, sliced and divided

Directions:

1. First, keep half of the banana, salt, oats, vanilla, cinnamon, almond milk, nutmeg, and maple syrup in the blender pitcher.
2. After that, press the 'cook' button and then the 'high' button.
3. Cook for 5 minutes.
4. Once done, divide the oatmeal among the serving bowls and top it with the remaining sliced banana and hempseeds.

Nutrition Info: Fat: 5.3 g Calories: 189 Total Carbs: 34.9 g Fiber: 7.5 g Sugar: 15.3 g Protein: 3.9 g Cholesterol: 0

Pork Carnitas

Servings: 6
Cooking Time: 3 Hours
Ingredients:

- Lime wedges
- 3 jalapeno pepper, minced
- A handful of cilantro, chopped
- 1 cup of chicken broth
- 2 Tbsp olive oil
- Corn tortilla
- 3lb pork shoulder, cut into cubes
- Queso Fresco, crumbled
- 2 Tbsp pork rubs

Directions:

1. Preheat wood pellet smoker-grill to 300^{0}F.
2. Mop the rub over the pork shoulder. Place pork shoulder in a cast-iron Dutch oven and pour in chicken broth. Transfer pot to grill grate and cook 2½ hours, until fork tender.
3. Remove the cover, bring to a boil then reduce the liquid in pot by half. All this happens within 15 minutes.
4. Place a tablespoon of bacon fat on the skillet and fry the pork for about 10 minutes, until crisp.
5. Take out pork and serve with cilantro, jalapeno, lime, queso fresco, and corn tortillas.

Nutrition Info: Per Serving: Calories: 254kcal, Carbs: 6g, Fat: 6g, Protein: 41g

Baked Wild Sockeye Salmon

Servings: 6
Cooking Time: 45 Minutes
Ingredients:
- 6 sockeye salmon fillets
- 3/4 tsp Old bay seasoning
- 1/2 tsp Seafood seasoning.

Directions:
1. Set the wood pellet smoker-grill to indirect cooking at 400 F
2. Rinse the fillet and pat dry with a paper towel. Add the seasoning, then rub all over the fillets.
3. Arrange fillets in a baking dish with the skin facing down, then transfer the dish to the cooking grid. Cover grill and bake for 15-20 minutes or until fillets begin to flake.
4. Serve.

Nutrition Info: Per Serving: Calories: 294kcal, Carbs: 10g, Fat:1g, Protein: 26g

Baby Bok Choy With Lime-miso Vinaigrette

Servings: 4
Cooking Time: 25 Minutes
Ingredients:
- ¼ cup good-quality vegetable oil
- Grated zest of 1 lime
- 2 tablespoons fresh lime juice
- 2 tablespoons white or light miso

- 1 tablespoon rice vinegar
- Salt and pepper
- 1½ pounds baby bok choy

Directions:
1. Start the coals or heat a gas grill for medium direct cooking. Make sure the grates are clean.
2. Whisk the oil, lime zest and juice, miso, and vinegar together in a small bowl until combined and thickened. Taste and adjust the seasoning with salt and pepper.
3. Trim the bottoms from the bok choy and cut into halves or quarters as needed. Pour half the vinaigrette into a large baking dish. Add the bok choy and turn in the vinaigrette until completely coated.
4. Put the bok choy on the grill directly over the fire. Close the lid and cook, turning once, until the leaves brown, and you can insert a knife through the core with no resistance, 5 to 10 minutes per side, depending on their size. Transfer to a platter, drizzle with the reserved vinaigrette and serve warm or at room temperature.

Nutrition Info: Calories: 209.7 Fats: 9.4 g Cholesterol: 7.4 mg Carbohydrates: 25.9 g Fiber: 4.5 g Sugars: 3 g Proteins: 10.1 g

Turkey Sandwich

Servings: 4
Cooking Time: 20 Minutes
Ingredients:
- 8 bread slices
- 1 cup gravy
- 2 cups turkey, cooked and shredded

Directions:
1. Set your wood pellet grill to smoke.
2. Preheat it to 400 degrees F.
3. Place a grill mat on top of the grates.
4. Add the turkey on top of the mat.
5. Cook for 10 minutes.
6. Toast the bread in the flame broiler.
7. Top the bread with the gravy and shredded turkey.

Nutrition Info: Calories: 280 Fat: 3.5 g Cholesterol: 20 mg Carbohydrates: 46 g Fiber: 5 g Sugars: 7 g Protein: 18 g

Smoked Spicy Pork Medallions

Servings: 6
Cooking Time: 1 Hour And 45 Minutes
Ingredients:
- 2 pounds pork medallions
- 3/4 cup chicken stock
- 1/2 cup tomato sauce (organic)
- 2 Tbs of smoked hot paprika (or to taste)
- 2 Tbsp of fresh basil finely chopped
- 1 Tbsp oregano
- Salt and pepper to taste

Directions:
1. Combine the chicken stock, tomato sauce, paprika, oregano, salt, and pepper.
2. Brush on tenderloin. Smoke grill for 4-5 minutes
3. Temperature must rise to 250 degrees Fahrenheit until 15 to 15 minutes at most
4. Place the pork on the grill grate and smoke until the internal temperature of the pork is at least medium-rare (about 145°F), for 1 1/2 hours.

Nutrition Info: Calories: 364.2 Cal Fat: 14.4 g Carbohydrates: 4 g Protein: 52.4 g Fiber: 2 g

Monster Smoked Pork Chops

Servings: 4
Cooking Time: 2 Hours 30 Minutes
Ingredients:
- 1/3 cup of sugar
- 4 tsp of pink curing salt
- Vegetable oil
- 1 cup of kosher or sea salt
- 1-1/4 pound pork chops
- 1/4 hot water
- 1/4 cold water

Directions:
1. Put the pork on a big baking pan. Mix the salt, curing salt, sugar, and hot water in a bowl. Add the pork to the mixture, and refrigerate for 12 hours.
2. Preheat the grill for 15 minutes at 250°F. Use pecan wood pellets
3. Bring the pork out and remove the brine from the pork.
4. Smoke the pork for about two and a half hours until it is done or until the internal temperature reads 145°F.
5. Brush olive oil all over the sides of the pork. Then increase the temperature of the cooker to 300°F and grill the pork chop for another 5 minutes until it is done.

Nutrition Info: Per Serving: Calories: 350kcal, Protein: 35g, Carbs: 45g, Fat: 40g.

APPENDIX : RECIPES INDEX

A

Apple Veggie Burger 9
Asian Steak Skewers 66
Authentic Holiday Turkey Breast 26
Avocado Smoothie 102

B

Baby Bok Choy With Lime-miso Vinaigrette 108
Bacon-wrapped Jalapeño Poppers 20
Bacon-wrapped Scallops 81
Bacon-wrapped Shrimp 75
Baked Parmesan Mushrooms 16
Baked Sweet And Savory Yams 22
Baked Wild Sockeye Salmon 108
Banana Nut Oatmeal 107
Banana Walnut Bread 104
Barbecue Sandwich 97
Bbq Baby Back Ribs 59
Bbq Breakfast Grits 67
Bbq Brisket 65
Bbq Sauce Smothered Chicken Breasts 44
Bbq Sweet Pepper Meatloaf 48
Beef Shoulder Clod 55
Beer Can Chicken 33
Beer Can–smoked Chicken 28
Black Bean Dipping Sauce 98
Braised Elk Shank 51
Braised Lamb 62
Braised Mediterranean Beef Brisket 69
Braised Short Ribs 67
Buffalo Chicken Flatbread 39
Buffalo Chicken Wraps 37
Buffalo Wings 45
Bunny Dogs With Sweet And Spicy Jalapeño Relish 9
Butter Braised Green Beans 23
Buttered Crab Legs 91
Buttered Green Peas 101
Buttered Thanksgiving Turkey 37

C

Cajun Catfish 83
Cajun Chicken 40
Cajun Seasoned Shrimp 87
Cajun Smoked Catfish 89
Cajun-blackened Shrimp 78
Caldereta Stew 10
Carolina Baked Beans 24

Charleston Crab Cakes With Remoulade 74
Chicken Wings 43
Chile Cheeseburgers 93
Chilean Sea Bass 88
Chili Barbecue Chicken 34
Chili Rib Eye Steaks 70
Chinese Bbq Pork 52
Chinese Inspired Duck Legs 41
Christmas Dinner Goose 30
Cider Salmon 82
Cinco De Mayo Chicken Enchiladas 39
Citrus Pork Chops 60
Citrus Salmon 75
Citrus-brined Pork Roast 54
Cocoa Crusted Pork Tenderloin 64
Coconut Bacon 21
Cod With Lemon Herb Butter 81
Cold Hot Smoked Salmon 94
Corn Chowder 24
Cornish Game Hens 98
Country Pork Roast 51
Cowboy Cut Steak 61
Cowboy Steak 53
Crazy Delicious Lobster Tails 85
Crispy & Juicy Chicken 31
Crispy Maple Bacon Brussels Sprouts 8
Cumin Salt 105
Curried Chicken Roast With Tarragon And Custard 94

D

Dijon-smoked Halibut 74
Drunken Beef Jerky 62

E

Easy Smoked Chicken Breasts 32
Elegant Lamb Chops 58
Empanadas 104
Enticing Mahi-mahi 86

F

Fish Fillets With Pesto 87
Flavor-bursting Prawn Skewers 78
French Onion Burgers 63

G

Garlic Aioli And Smoked Salmon Sliders 96
Garlic And Herb Smoke Potato 15
Garlic And Rosemary Potato Wedges 12
Garlic Parmesan Chicken Wings 33

Garlic Rack Of Lamb 56
Georgia Sweet Onion Bake 19
Glazed Chicken Thighs 26
Greek-style Roast Leg Of Lamb 70
Grilled Asparagus & Honey-glazed Carrots 23
Grilled Asparagus With Wild Mushrooms 6
Grilled Bacon Dog 100
Grilled Blackened Salmon 76
Grilled Broccoli 21
Grilled Cherry Tomato Skewers 19
Grilled Corn On The Cob With Parmesan And Garlic 14
Grilled Cuban Pork Chops 55
Grilled King Crab Legs 83
Grilled Lingcod 84
Grilled Lobster Tail 90
Grilled Rainbow Trout 87
Grilled Ratatouille Salad 11
Grilled Salmon 86
Grilled Shrimp 89
Grilled Shrimp Kabobs 77
Grilled Shrimp Scampi 79
Grilled Tilapia 78
Grilled Tuna 86
Grilled Zucchini Squash 16
Grilled Zucchini Squash Spears 17

H

Halibut With Garlic Pesto 90
Herb Roasted Turkey 27
Hickory Smoked Chicken 35
Hickory Smoked Chicken Leg And Thigh Quarters 45
Hickory Smoked Green Beans 103
Honey Garlic Chicken Wings 34
Hot And Sweet Spatchcocked Chicken 46
Hot-smoked Salmon 90

J

Jamaican Jerk Chicken Quarters 30
Jerk Shrimp 87
Juicy Smoked Salmon 75

K

Kalbi Beef Ribs 63
Kale Chips 12

L

Lamb Shank 58
Lemon Chicken Breast 27
Lemon Garlic Scallops 76

Lemon Rosemary And Beer Marinated Chicken 26
Lively Flavored Shrimp 80
Lobster Tail 72
Lobster Tails 73

M

Mango Shrimp 89
Maple And Bacon Chicken 44
Mesquite Smoked Brisket 58
Mexican Street Corn With Chipotle Butter 2 18
Minestrone Soup 16
Monster Smoked Pork Chops 109
Mussels With Pancetta Aïoli 84

N

Native Southern Cornbread 101
No-fuss Tuna Burgers 83

O

Omega-3 Rich Salmon 85
Oysters In The Shell 77

P

Pacific Northwest Salmon 77
Pan-seared Pork Tenderloin With Apple Mashed Potatoes 102
Paprika Chicken 42
Peach And Basil Grilled Chicken 27
Peppered Bbq Chicken Thighs 30
Perfectly Smoked Turkey Legs 42
Pineapple Pork Bbq 50
Pineapple-pepper Pork Kebabs 57
Pizza Bianca 97
Polish Kielbasa 99
Pork Belly 50
Pork Carnitas 107
Pork Fennel Burger 99
Pork Steak 49
Potato Fries With Chipotle Peppers 15
Potluck Favorite Baked Beans 105

R

Ramen Soup 7
Real Treat Chuck Roast 53
Red Wine Beef Stew 106
Reverse Seared Flank Steak 49
Reverse-seared Tilapia 98
Roasted Almonds 100
Roasted Butternut Squash 15
Roasted Ham 98
Roasted Hasselback Potatoes 9

Roasted Okra 18
Roasted Parmesan Cheese Broccoli 10
Roasted Peach Salsa 7
Roasted Root Vegetables 13
Roasted Spicy Tomatoes 20
Roasted Vegetable Medley 24
Roasted Veggies & Hummus 17
Roasted Whole Chicken 33
Rosemary Lamb 68
Rosemary Orange Chicken 28
Rustic Maple Smoked Chicken Wings 41

S

Salmon With Avocado Salsa 85
Salt-crusted Baked Potatoes 19
Santa Maria Tri-tip 71
Seafaring Seafood Rub With Smoked Swordfish 106
Seafood On Skewers 95
Seared Tuna Steaks 91
Shiitake Smoked Mushrooms 20
Slow Roasted Shawarma 61
Smo-fried Chicken 29
Smoked 3-bean Salad 8
Smoked And Pulled Beef 53
Smoked And Smashed New Potatoes 23
Smoked Baked Beans 11
Smoked Baked Kale Chips 21
Smoked Balsamic Potatoes And Carrots 11
Smoked Bananas Foster Bread Pudding 95
Smoked Cheese Dip 93
Smoked Chicken With Perfect Poultry Rub 96
Smoked Chuck Roast 94
Smoked Deviled Eggs 12
Smoked Eggs 21
Smoked Fried Chicken 39
Smoked Garlic White Sauce 96
Smoked Healthy Cabbage 7
Smoked Lamb Meatballs 66
Smoked Lemon Chicken Breasts 38
Smoked Longhorn Cowboy Tri-tip 68
Smoked Mushrooms 22
Smoked Pork Ribs With Fresh Herbs 93
Smoked Pork Sausages 54
Smoked Pork Tenderloin 64
Smoked Potato Salad 17
Smoked Pumpkin Soup 13
Smoked Sausages 65

Smoked Shrimp 76
Smoked Spicy Pork Medallions 109
Smoked Teriyaki Tuna 103
Smoked Tuna 106
Smoked Turkey Breast 32
Smoked Turkey Wings 35
Smoked Whole Duck 43
Smoked, Candied, And Spicy Bacon 57
Smokey Roasted Cauliflower 22
Smoking Duck With Mandarin Glaze 38
Southern Slaw 6
Southern Sugar-glazed Ham 60
Spatchcocked Turkey 45
Special Occasion's Dinner Cornish Hen 29
Spiced Nuts 100
Spicy & Tangy Lamb Shoulder 62
Spicy Shrimps Skewers 91
Spinach Soup 6
Sriracha Salmon 72
St. Louis Bbq Ribs 48
Steak Sauce 101
Strip Steak With Onion Sauce 55
Stuffed Grilled Zucchini 23
Stuffed Shrimp Tilapia 73
Stunning Prime Rib Roast 60
Summer Paella 81
Super-addicting Mushrooms 99
Super-tasty Trout 77
Sweet & Spicy Pork Roast 59
Sweet And Spicy Smoked Wings 40
Sweet Potato Chips 14
Sweet Potato Fries 18
Sweet Sensation Pork Meat 103
Sweet Smoked Country Ribs 64

T

Teriyaki Smoked Shrimp 88
Texas Smoked Brisket 52
The Perfect T-bones 48
Togarashi Smoked Salmon 72
Asian Miso Chicken Wings 32
Bacon 66
Beef Jerky 57
Fries With Chipotle Ketchup 13
Grill Bbq Chicken Breasts 31
Grilled Buffalo Chicken Legs 36
Grilled Chicken 42
Grilled Lingcod 80

Lobster Tail 80
Marinated Chicken Kabobs 105
Salmon With Togarashi 80
Sheet Pan Chicken Fajitas 41
Smoked Pork Ribs 68
Smoked Shrimp 85
Stuffed Peppers 69
Trager New York Strip 50
Turkey Breast 40
Turkey Meatballs 38
Turkey Sandwich 108
Turkey With Apricot Barbecue Glaze 43
Twice-baked Spaghetti Squash 102

V

Vegan Smoked Carrot Dogs 8
Versatile Beef Tenderloin 56

W

Whole Roasted Cauliflower With Garlic Parmesan Butter 20
Wild Turkey Egg Rolls 36
Wild West Wings 46
Wine Infused Salmon 79
Wood Pellet Bacon Wrapped Jalapeno Poppers 11
Wood Pellet Chicken Breasts 36
Wood Pellet Chile Lime Chicken 45
Wood Pellet Garlic Dill Smoked Salmon 88

Wood Pellet Grill Pork Crown Roast 68
Wood Pellet Grilled Asparagus And Honey Glazed Carrots 6
Wood Pellet Grilled Buffalo Chicken Leg 34
Wood Pellet Grilled Chicken 35
Wood Pellet Grilled Lamb With Brown Sugar Glaze 65
Wood Pellet Grilled Shredded Pork Tacos 53
Wood Pellet Rockfish 82
Wood Pellet Salt And Pepper Spot Prawn Skewers 79
Wood Pellet Sheet Pan Chicken Fajitas 32
Wood Pellet Smoked Acorn Squash 17
Wood Pellet Smoked Asparagus 8
Wood Pellet Smoked Cornish Hens 44
Wood Pellet Smoked Leg Of lamb 49
Wood Pellet Smoked Salmon 92
Wood Pellet Smoked Spatchcock Turkey 29
Wood Pellet Smoked Spatchcock Turkey 34
Wood Pellet Smoked Vegetables 14
Wood Pellet Spicy Brisket 107
Wood Pellet Teriyaki Smoked Shrimp 83
Wood Pellet Togarashi Grilled Salmon 74
Wood Pellet Togarashi Pork Tenderloin 51
Wood-fired Chicken Breasts 46

CPSIA information can be obtained
at www.ICGtesting.com
Printed in the USA
LVHW061605260621
691218LV00009B/924